Squeezed Middle: Mental Health in Decline

Vani

Table of Contents

Chapter 1

Introduction

Over the past several decades, the United States has witnessed growing

inequality, decreasing wages, and increasing instability in work (Krugman, 2012; Stiglitz,

2015). A shrinking middle class and disengaged workforce are urgent public health

concerns in light of the Commission of Social Determinants of Health's declaration that

low socioeconomic status (SES) is one the strongest predictors of mental and physical

well-being (Solar & Irwin, 2018), and the growing body of research documenting the link

between work and mental health (Paul & Moser, 2009; Swanson, 2012). Coupled with

these economic shifts, rapid advances in technology and expanding globalization have led

to a dissipating low-skill labor market, impacting those with limited education and

resources the hardest (Benzell, Kotlikoff, LaGarda, & Sachs, 2015; OECD, 2015). The

2020 COVID-19 pandemic has further exacerbated these work-based uncertainties and

inequities, and exposed vulnerabilities to securing decent work for individuals from

marginalized backgrounds (BLS, 2020; ILO, 2020). Despite the breadth of research

documenting links between work and well-being, studies rarely attend to community

factors that shape opportunity for accessing work. Hence, exploring relationships among

declining decent work and mental health within and across various geographic locations

is of critical importance according to a social justice agenda.

Despite increasing knowledge of the importance of contextual factors in the

development and psychological well-being of humans (Bronfenbrenner & Morris, 2006),

psychology has been slow to move beyond individual-level investigations. MacLachlan

(2014) argues that this neglect is due to psychology's failure to move beyond traditional approaches of studies on an individual-level and removed from context, such as laboratory setting. Conversely, economists have made strides in examining ways that political and economic forces shape opportunity structures, and how these conditions impact individuals' capacities to engage in meaningful work (Nussbaum, 2011; Sen, 1999). Additionally, occupational sociologists have examined relationships among multi-level factors, such as labor markets, organizational policies, and individual experiences of work (e.g., Kalleberg, 2009; Kalleberg & Vallas, 2017). Capitalizing on these fields' promising and holistic efforts, counseling psychology research driven by innovative techniques and interdisciplinary approaches may capture a more realistic understanding of peoples' work lives, which occur in various contexts.

While MacLachlan's (2014) charge is relevant across the vast array psychological fields, some vocational psychologists have similarly upheld this mission and crafted a transformative, social-justice informed, vocational psychology agenda, expanding beyond individual career decision-making to address work-related issues impacting those with limited volition, such as unemployment, underemployment, precarious work, and access to decent work (Blustein, Ali, & Flores, 2019). By acknowledging greater economic, political, and technological forces, these vocational scholars harken for the inclusion of knowledge from these disciplines into future research on work-related issues. Demonstrating enormous progress in advancing understanding of individuals' work lives, numerous vocational psychologists committed to a social justice agenda place community conditions as the premiere determinant of access to decent work (Ali et al., 2017; Flores et al., 2017). Not only are communities crucial in shaping work opportunities, aggregate individual employment and/or job loss have enormous implications for the health and livelihood of communities (Abramovitz & Albercht, 2013; Ali et al., 2017; Wilson, 2017). Following this logic, systemic interventions at a community level may arguably best promote individuals' work lives and well-being amidst the drastically changing work landscape, particularly for traditionally marginalized populations (Ali, 2013; Blustein, 2008; Solberg & Ali, 2017). Given the overwhelming research documenting negative health consequences of inequality and unemployment coupled with lack of research on community-level factors, the present study explored the role of community opportunity on individuals' work lives across the geographic diversity of the United States in order to inform public policy and community-specific interventions.

The Psychology of Working

Vocational psychology has advanced increasingly inclusive theoretical frameworks over the past several decades, which have been instrumental in supporting career decision-making and development for people and in fostering work satisfaction and well-being (Blustein, 2006; 2013). Despite these foundational works in the field (e.g., Holland, 1997; Lent, 2013), they have proven primarily applicable to people with a degree of choice in their work lives. To remedy the exclusion of those from marginalized backgrounds with limited work volition, Blustein proposed the Psychology of Working Framework (PWF; 2006) to assert the fundamental role of work in meeting individuals' basic and psychological needs, the interwoven nature of work and non-work domains, the need for greater attention to the changing world of work, and the inclusion of "all those who work and desire to work". The PWF perspective (Blustein, 2006; 2008), along with an empirically testable Psychology of Working Theory (PWT; Duffy et al., 2016),

considers the contextual factors of marginalization and economic constraints as the

primary predictors of access to decent work and subsequent vocational and psychological

well-being. Given its primacy in determining well-being, the International Labor

Organization (ILO; 2008) considers decent work to be a basic human right and defines it

as work that offers adequate compensation, safe working conditions and protection

against unemployment.

According to PWT (Duffy et al., 2016), the pathways from marginalization (e.g.

experiences of identity-based discrimination) and economic constraints (i.e. limited

financial resources and social capital) to decent work are mediated by work volition, or

the perception of choice in career decision-making (Duffy, Diemer, Perry, Laurenzi, &

Torrey, 2012). PWT theorists initially posited that attaining decent work fulfills three

essential human needs: survival (i.e. financial means), relatedness (i.e. social connection

with others), and self-determination (i.e. asserting one's identity and agency), and have

since expanded on these needs through empirical testing to encompass five needs:

survival, social contribution, autonomy, competence, and relatedness (Autin et al., 2019).

Fulfillment of these needs then is positively associated with life and job satisfaction.

Along with hypothesized direct and indirect pathways, PWT proposes several possible

moderators in the paths from marginalization and economic constraints to work volition,

and from marginalization and economic constraints to decent work (Duffy et al., 2016).

The proposed moderator of economic conditions represents forces outside of individuals'

immediate environments, such as economic trends and unemployment rates, and may

contribute to the study's aim to understand vocational and psychological health in the context of the current economic and political climate. Furthermore, the PWT model is particularly relevant to this study, which sought to incorporate communities where economic conditions are declining and opportunities for decent work are disappearing; this study also embodies an intersectional lens to capture the reality that people may experience multiple forms of oppression that accumulate and interact in complex ways (Cho, Crenshaw, & McCall, 2013).

Since its inception, PWT has spurred a steadily growing empirical base, both domestically and internationally. Researchers have most frequently explored how the contextual predictor variables and proposed mediators relate to decent work. Notably, support for the proposition of economic constraints directly predicting access to decent work has remained inconclusive (Douglass, Velez, Conlin, Duffy, England, 2017; Duffy et al., 2017; Duffy et al., 2019; see Blustein & Duffy, in press for a full review). To rule out mis-specification of the economic constraints construct as a possible cause for the tenet's mixed findings, the present study incorporated objective social class and current and childhood subjective social class, as indicators of the construct. Furthermore, although PWT scholars conceptualize decent work as a multidimensional construct containing both a general construct and distinct subcomponents which comprise the global factor, the majority of research thus far has examined predictors and outcomes using a global construct (Douglass, Velez, Conlin, Duffy, England, 2017; Duffy et al., 2017; Duffy et al., 2019; see Blustein & Duffy, in press for a full review). Therefore, the present study aimed to expand understanding of the multidimensionality of work by examining its discrete components.

Along with an in-depth exploration of subcomponents of decent work and economic constraints, and their respective influences on work and well-being, the current study endeavored to expand upon knowledge of work volition by investigating the theorized moderation effect of economic conditions (Duffy et al., 2016). Although PWT scholars theorize that economic conditions will moderate pathways from predictor variables to decent work and from these variables to mediator variables by buffering against the negative impact of economic constraints and marginalization, they limit their discussion of possible economic condition variables mainly to unemployment rates and job growth rates (Duffy et al., 2016). Amid growing bodies of literature highlighting the negative and complex effects of community economic conditions, such as economic hardship, inequality, and unemployment rates, on access to work and well-being (Cheng & Lucas, 2016; Monnat & Brown, 2018; Muramotsa, 2003), the study addressed numerous potential indicators of economic conditions, honing in on conditions at a local level, as well expanding to community factors associated with economic conditions, such as education and youth engagement. Some research has demonstrated that economic inequality, rather than absolute poverty, has a greater negative impact on individual well-being (Diemer, Mistry, Wadsworth, López, & Reimers, 2013; Fine, Stoudt, Fox, & Santos, 2010). Given disparate findings related to indicators of economic conditions, the study attempted to illuminate which indicators have the greatest impact on work and life well-being. Along with economic conditions, a breadth of literature has found that factors, such as education and engaged youth, are some of the strongest predictors of social mobility (Opportunity Nation & Measure of America, 2017). Yet, limited research has explored the impact of these forms of community opportunity on individual work outcomes. Therefore, the current study expands on PWT scholars' hypothesis of the importance economic conditions by conceptualizing it as one form of opportunity and exploring other forms of community opportunity as well.

Exploring community economic conditions and community opportunity more broadly holds promise considering work volition's association with numerous positive work outcomes, as well as theoretical assumptions that work volition is shaped by real structural barriers (Blustein, 2006, 2008; Duffy et al., 2012). Thus, various indicators of community opportunity, and/or lack thereof, may act as structural barriers to individuals in pursuit of decent work. Because work volition is a psychological construct, community conditions, such as inequality and unemployment rates, may shape its formation, consistent with findings demonstrating their negative influence on mental health, as hypothesized by relative deprivation and social comparison theories (Festinger, 1954; Fine et al., 2010).

Thus, the current study explored the PWT-theorized direct pathway from social class, measured both objectively and subjectively to decent work, and indirectly from social class to decent work via work volition. Secondly, the study investigated how predictors related to the five discrete components of decent work, in conjunction with a global factor, and whether decent work predicted life satisfaction. Furthermore, the study explored potential moderation effects of economic conditions and other forms of opportunity on the pathways from social class to work volition, as well as the path from predictor variables to well-being, as measured by overall life satisfaction.

To test these proposed pathways, the study employed structural equation modeling (SEM) with a national adult sample, geographically representative of the US population. Analyses involved matching individual participant data to their county-specific opportunity data (Opportunity Nation & Measure of America, 2017). Following an in-depth review of literature, this book will detail the study's methodology and analytic approach. The next chapter will present results of hypotheses testing, and the final chapter will conclude with a discussion of results, study limitations, and implications for research, theoretical, practice, and policy.

Chapter 2

Literature Review

Evidence of the impact of work on psychological health is vast, as is its role in upward mobility and/or maintaining systemic oppression (Blustein, 2006; 2008; Lent, 2004; Swanson, 2012). Work has the potential to foster mental well-being by connecting individuals to broader society and providing a source of individual accomplishment (Blustein, 2008); relatedly research has documented numerous consequences related to job loss and unemployment, including anxiety, low self-esteem, and substance abuse, among other deleterious effects (Blustein, 2008; Vinokur et al., 2000). As mentioned previously, decent work not only asserts a powerful influence on individual well-being, but also on the potential for upward mobility in communities, as well as other markers of community health, such as crime rates and educational attainment (Abramovitz & Albercht, 2013; Ali et al., 2017; Wilson, 2017).

Further testament to the powerful role of work in individuals' lives is evident in the ILO's declaration of decent work as a human right (ILO, 2008/2012). However, the ILO has concurrently attested to declining access to decent work (2008/2012), along with social scientists across disciplines highlighting the interplay among work, economics, and technology, in exacerbating social inequality (Picketty, 2014; Stiglitz, 2015). For instance, Katz attested to struggles of working-class populations, previously employed in manufacturing, as they must adapt to work landscape shifts, such as increasing levels of automation and technology use (2011). Similarly, prominent occupational sociologists have cited occupational polarization as a major contributor to increasing economic inequality rates (e.g., Mouw & Kalleberg, 2010; Vallas, 2011), such that although "high skill" jobs are increasing as a result of technological advances and globalization, middle skills jobs are shrinking, intensifying wage discrepancies. Marginalized groups primarily focused on making ends meet are most susceptible to experiencing precariousness (Kalleberg, 2009; Standing, 2010). The COVID-19 crisis has exemplified the polarity of precarious work in that many of those with "high skill" jobs have been able to continue working remotely, whereas those in contract work or "low skill" jobs have been more likely to be laid off or face potentially unsafe working conditions (ILO, 2020). Precarious work entails work that is short-term, often contract based, and lacks security (Kalleberg, 2009; Kalleberg & Vallas, 2017). While human development economists have emphasized the potential for individuals in poverty to assert their agency in moving toward work and increasing well-being (Nussbaum, 2011; Roberston, 2015; Sen, 1999), poor economic conditions and oppressive structures can limit individuals' ability to assert their agency and take action. To this end, Guichard (2013) aptly called for the inclusion of decent work in vocational psychology's agenda to promote social justice.

While the ILO (2012) outlines guidelines for improving access to decent work through policy changes and involvement in the labor market, research has demonstrated the need to better understand individuals' psychological experiences of work and how they construct meaning of these experiences (Blustein, Olle, Connors-Kellgren, & Diamonti, 2016). One of the outcomes of recent attention in psychology to the ILO's work is the construction of a decent work scale to integrate contextual and individual psychological variables in order to capture a realistic understanding of work experiences for marginalized groups (Duffy et al., 2016; Duffy et al., 2017). Furthermore, PWT encourages researchers to investigate the "interplay between contextual, psychological, and economic factors" and has recommended integrating individual self-reports with broader macrolevel indicators outlined by the ILO, such as unemployment rates and union density (Duffy et al., 2016; ILO, 2012). Accordingly, the present study sought to better understand relationships among individuals' contextual factors and work-related psychological constructs, in conjunction with community economic conditions, and access to decent work, as measured by meeting the five components of decent work: safe working conditions, adequate compensation, access to healthcare, adequate rest and free time, and a match of organizational and social/family values (Duffy et al., 2016; Duffy et al., 2017).

To frame the current study, the literature review first explores empirical support and limitations for the PWT model related to the contextual predicator variable of economic constraints, focusing specifically on the conceptualization of this construct as social class variables in the PWT model. Next, the review attends to the measurement of, and empirical findings related to, decent work. The following section introduces work volition as a construct, and the potential influence of community economic conditions on its formation. To this end, the subsequent section attends to instances of contextual factors, such as economic trends and geographical location, impacting psychological and vocational well-being through impact on community economic conditions. Within this domain, the review attends to the role economic inequality plays in shaping individual psychological experiences, given the increasing wealth gap in the US (Picketty, 2014; Standing, 2010). Final sections integrate research on social capital and well-being to highlight potential ways that community economic conditions and opportunity may disrupt community well-being and individual outcomes.

Empirical Support for PWT

Predictor Variables

Given the role of work in social mobility, the impetus of PWF was largely to include individuals from poor and working-class backgrounds in career development research, theory, and interventions to address this population's limited access to decent work and accompanying persistent marginalization (Blustein, 2006, 2008). Social class plays a major role in shaping work opportunities, which confer varying levels of prestige and financial rewards, and subsequently contribute to the maintenance of social class (Diemer & Ali, 2009). Therefore, work may act as the major mechanism maintaining intergenerational poverty (Wagmiller & Adelman, 2009). In addition to lacking resources for career development, those living in poverty are likely mainly focused on immediate problems of survival and thus unable to devote time and energy toward more long-term goals (Shah, Mullainathan, & Shafir, 2012). Relatedly, a breadth of research has explored associations among social class, career development, and work-related outcomes, demonstrating its relationship to beliefs about locus of control and ability in the work settings, lower outcome expectations, less self-efficacy in career decision-making, lower job satisfaction, and to career aspirations associated with less prestige (Brown et al., 1996; Perry & Wallace, 2013; Metheny & McWhirter; 2013; Thompson & Dahling, 2010). Although PWT scholars acknowledge the complexity of studying economic constraints and marginalization, citing theory on intersectionality (Cole, 2009; Purdie-Vaughns & Eibach, 2008), they conceptualize them as distinct but related constructs in the PWT model (Duffy et al., 2016). For example, authors note that marginalization from social identities may impede individuals' ability to utilize available economic resources (Duffy et al., 2016). Accordingly, an individual's objective social class, or available economic resources and social capital (Krieger, Williams, & Moss, 1996), relates to access to decent work, as well as class-related marginalization, resulting from perceptions of social class or their power and influence in society, namely subjective social class (Krieger et al., 1996).

Extant studies utilizing the PWT model have used both objective and subjective measures of social class as measures of economic constraints (Blustein et al., under review; Douglass et al., 2017; Duffy et al., 2018; Duffy, Gensmer et al., 2019). Despite a breadth of empirical support for the association between economic constraints and marginalization, several initial studies using PWT did not yield support for this proposition (Douglass et al., 2017; Duffy et al., 2018). While a breadth of research has demonstrated indirect relationships between predictor variables and decent work via work volition (Douglass et al., 2017; Duffy et al., 2018; Duffy, Gensmer et al., 2019; England et al., 2020), several studies have failed to lend support for the proposed direct pathway from economic constraints to decent work (Duffy, Gensmer et al., 2019). Given the critical role of social class in research on work-related outcomes (Ali et al., 2013), further investigation of both the availability of economic resources (objective social class) and class marginalization (subjective social status) is warranted.

Although research has demonstrated strong associations between objective and subjective measures of social class, they make unique contributions to access to decent work according to PWT (Diemer et al., 2013; Duffy et al., 2016; Krieger et al.,1997; Perry & Wallace, 2013). Objective measures of socioeconomic status, such as income and educational attainment, convey important information regarding access to economic resources, which may constrain or facilitate pathways to decent work. Additionally, subjective measures of social class represent psychological experiences associated with contextual variables that influence an individual's ability to utilize their resources. Considering their interwoven nature, the present study will avoid artificial distinctions between economic constraints and class marginalization (Duffy et al., 2016) by examining the structure of a social class latent construct, incorporating both objective and subjective indicators.

The present study will thus employ both objective and subjective measures of social class that have been used extensively in research. Income will be used as an objective measure of social class, as scholars have recommended this indicator for cross-national comparisons and for making policy recommendations (Diemer et al., 2013; Roosa, Deng, Nair, & Burrell, 2005). Asking respondents to indicate which social class they belong to (e.g. poor, working class, middle class, etc.) communicates internalization of social class and will serve as a measure of subjective social status (Adler, Epel, Castellazzo, & Ickovics, 2000; Diemer et al., 2013). Duffy et al. (2019) emphasize the importance of assessing individuals' experience of economic constraints over their lifetime, given that access to resources in childhood influences career development and later occupational attainment. Therefore, the present study will ask participants to indicate their childhood social class as well.

Vocational psychologists have made strides in research with poor and working-class populations in recent years (Ali et al., 2013; Diemer & Ali, 2009; Perry & Wallace, 2013). While empirical studies on PWT have begun to explore marginalization and economic constraints, the complexity of studying social class (Perry & Wallace, 2013) warrants further research to inform the conceptualization of these constructs within the PWT model. Therefore, the present study will examine the link between social class and decent work via the mediator of work volition, as well as its direct link from social class to life satisfaction. While the PWT model does not include a hypothesized direct pathway from social class to life satisfaction, it implies a pathway through several variables, including work volition, decent work, and PWT needs (Duffy et al., 2016). Considering well-documented links between social class and well-being (Solar & Irwin, 2018), the current study sought to draw attention to this potential association within the PWT model.

Decent Work

As previously mentioned, PWT positions decent work as both a major outcome of contextual predictors and work volition, and as an antecedent to job and life satisfaction via its potential to satisfy essential needs (Duffy et al., 2016). To further measurement of decent work within the PWT model, researchers developed the Decent Work Scale (DWS) (Duffy et al., 2017). Scale developers proposed and tested three models for measuring decent work. In a hierarchical structure, the five components of DW are additive and when combined, comprise a higher-order global DW factor. In a correlational structure, the five components remain independent, without inclusion of a global factor. Finally, the bifactor structure measures the five independent components and a separate global factor, both portions which function synchronously (Duffy et al., 2017). Although scale developers recommend using the bifactor structure, several studies have found equivalent, if not slightly better, fit to the data when using the correlational structure (Buyukgoze-Kavas & Autin, 2019; Ferreira et al., 2019; see Kim et al., 2020 for a full review). Despite promising evidence for the correlational structure, most studies have tested hypothesized pathways with other variables in the full model using a global decent factor (Duffy, Gensmer et al., 2019; England et al., 2020). Although use of the global factor is beneficial when trying to understand the generality of DW, further research is needed to better understand how the distinct components of decent work function. While some research has examined the specificity of DW conditions through profile analyses (Blustein et al., under review; Kim et al.; 2020), no known studies have tested hypothesized pathways with the individual components of DW. Thus, the present study investigated the role of discrete components in the overall model, while also accounting for the presence of a global DW factor. (Buyukgoze-Kavas & Autin, 2019; Ferreira et al., 2019; see Kim et al., 2020 for a full review)

Work volition as mediator

A centerpiece of the PWF is the inclusion of people with limited work volition as a result of economic constraints and marginalization (Blustein, 2006). For these individuals, the primacy of meeting survival needs shapes career choice, potentially limiting the ability to choose work that is intrinsically motivating and satisfying (Blustein, 2006; 2008). Namely, barriers resulting from oppression based on race/ethnicity, gender, social class, sexual orientation, and a lack of resources may lead to low work volition, which in turn impacts access to work that also meets social contribution and self-determination needs and subsequent job satisfaction (Blustein, Kenna, Gill, & Devoy, 2008).

Originally theorized as a psychological construct shaped by structural and financial constraints, scholars have since developed measures of work volition, or the perception of choice in career decision-making (Duffy et al., 2012). Attending to the importance of both actual constraints and feelings of volition (Blustein et al., 2008), these researchers explored perceptions of a host of common career barriers (Blustein 2006, 2008; Blustein, McWhirter, & Perry, 2005) and more generally a sense of control and volition to determine a three-factor structure of work volition composed of volition, financial constraints, and structural constraints (Duffy et al., 2012). While researchers found correlations between career barriers and work volition, they determined that work volition contributed unique variance, above and beyond variance attributable to common predictors of work-related outcome variables, such as job satisfaction. As a result, researchers theorized that career barriers represent actual constraints, whereas work volition indicates a subjective experience (Duffy et al., 2012). In subsequent studies exploring this conceptualization of work volition, researchers found that career barriers and social class were predictors of work volition but also that work volition predicted a sense of control and career barriers (Duffy et al., 2016). These findings suggest that work volition may influence perceptions of future career barriers, and therefore, while predictors like social class are not malleable, work volition might act as an attitude that can be influenced, in addition to an outcome of actual barriers. Given promising findings on associations between work volition and positive vocational outcomes, work volition may prove facilitative for disadvantaged populations navigating to access decent work (Duffy, Douglass, & Autin, 2015). Therefore, PWT scholars have explored work volition as a major mediating variable between economic constraints and marginalization, and access to decent work.

Thus, a body of research has begun to test proposed mediated pathways to decent work in the PWT model. Studies that have focused on sexual and racial/ethnic minority populations have found support for indirect relationships from economic constraints and marginalization to decent work via work volition (Douglass et al., 2017; Duffy et al., 2018; Duffy et al., 2019; England et al., 2020). More specifically, work volition was positively associated with access to decent work, whereas economic constraints and marginalization were negatively associated with work volition in these mediated relationships.

Further exploration of work volition as a mechanism in accessing work opportunities may yield greater understanding of how this construct is influenced by social class, considering the breadth of research supporting its contribution to accessing decent work (Douglass et al., 2017; Duffy et al., 2018; Duffy et al., 2019). Furthermore, some conceptualizations of work volition have suggested that it is a mutable psychological asset, offering counseling psychologists a point of intervention (Duffy et al., 2012; Duffy et al., 2016). However, this line of research has explored predictors and outcomes of work volition using individual self-report measures of career barriers. Considering that research has demonstrated that individuals of varying class backgrounds report similar numbers of career barriers, albeit different types (Swanson, Daniels, & Tokar, 1996), work volition may not function similarly for all individuals, depending on the type and extent of the barriers they face. Therefore, research incorporating actual barriers in its design is necessary. While it may seem plausible to influence an individual's perception of volition, this may not suffice in environments with very limited opportunities for decent work. The present study thus explored the potential role of community opportunity as an indicator of actual structural barriers in understanding perceptions of work volition.

The previous sections have demonstrated promising findings related to the variables of social class and work volition in predicting access to decent work and the mediating the relationship, respectively (Douglass et al., 2017; Duffy et al., 2018; Duffy et al., 2019). However, given that empirical research on the PWT model is in its infancy, additional research is needed to hone predictor constructs, in this case integrating both objective and subjective social class into a latent construct, and incorporating community opportunity and barriers in the investigation of social position variables and work volition. The following sections will thus explore the proposed moderator of economic conditions that have not yet been tested in the PWT model, and offer a means to integrate structural barriers in examining intersections of social position variables, work-related psychological constructs, access to decent work and life satisfaction.

Community and the Individual

Although researchers in psychological fields have historically struggled to link micro and macro-level factors in study designs (MacLachlan, 2014), work volition presents an opportunity to explore this link given its conceptualization as an individual psychological construct that is, in part, shaped by structural barriers. Thus, the present study conceptualizes community opportunity as structural barriers that influence perceptions and constrains opportunities, in this case related to career choice. Community opportunity is a robust variable, spanning domains of economic, civic engagement, education, and health (Opportunity Nation & Measure of America, 2017). Community unemployment rates may appear most relevant as a structural factor that impacts individual development of work volition, as well as other dimensions of community opportunity, such as educational attainment and youth. However, education and civic engagement may also influence work volition, considering the role of education in career development and access to career opportunities, as well as studies documenting associations of disconnected youth and overall community opportunity, all which contribute to the climate in which real access to decent work and associated psychological outcomes derive (Lewis, 2019). Therefore, the discussion of community factors and individual work and psychological outcomes will begin by assessing the role of economic conditions and expand to incorporate additional forms of community opportunity. Given their inextricable links, the following sections will explore the role of community in several individual outcomes, including social mobility, physical and mental health, and work outcomes.

To begin, the review will provide evidence of ways in which community and individuals are shaped historically by economic trends, such as recessions, prior to highlighting critical variations in the impact of these trends according to geographic location. The subsequent section will explore more specific dimensions of community economic conditions, including poverty and unemployment rates, while attending most to economic inequality considering that theories of social comparison and relative deprivation elucidate its potential to shape individual perceptions, such as work volition (Festinger, 1954; Kawachi et al., 1998). Finally, the review will utilize social capital theory (Coleman & Coleman, 1994; Kawachi et al., 1998; Putnam, 2000) as a lens by which to further extrapolate how individual perceptions and outcomes are formed by various opportunities and dynamics in communities, thus necessitating integrative analyses of individual, community, and geographic factors. Consistent with PWT's interdisciplinary theoretical underpinnings (Duffy et al., 2016), the literature review on community and the individual draws from several disciplines in attempts to fully capture the complexity of access to decent work and its outcomes, including economics, epidemiology and public health, and sociology, among others, in addition to various psychological fields.

Economic Trends

Historical Context. Ties between economic trends and individual livelihoods are evident as economists have noted that intergenerational upward mobility has declined throughout the 20th century (Chetty et al., 2016). Although the US Gross Domestic Product (GDP) has increased since the 1940s, researchers have demonstrated that absolute income, compared to one's parents, dropped from a 90 percent increase in the 1940s to a 50 percent increase in the 1980s and 1990s. Economists thus attribute declining upward mobility to the uneven distribution of GDP, and this decline has important implications for individual mental and physical health, given that SES represents one of the most robust social determinants of health (Solar & Irwin, 2018). The ensuing section seeks to illuminate the interplay among economic trends, work, and well-being.

In the aftermath of the Great Recession (2007 – 2009), social scientists mobilized to understand the impact of a national and global economic trauma on well-being. A meta-analysis examining economic recessions and mental health suggests links between economic and mental health declines across the globe (Frasquilho, 2016). The study revealed associations between unemployment rates at both macro and individual levels and mental illness diagnoses, including suicidal behavior, thus conveying the financial and psychological costs in response to national and global economic crises. A closer look at the US context specifically indicates that suicides in the year immediately following the financial cash (2008-2009) were correlated with unemployment at the county level, but that the relationship was mediated by county poverty levels (Kerr et al., 2017). Bearing in mind the enormous cost to human life, psychologists must integrate economic declines and collapses into their conceptualizations of the development of mental illness and attend to specific US communities that may be at risk due to poor economic conditions.

Geographic Context. Along with exemplifying economic shifts historically, economists have demonstrated significant geographic variation in these trends, such as differing upward mobility, with regions in the Southeast US representing the lowest increases and regions in the Mountain and Pacific regions demonstrating the greatest growth, with median rates occurring in the New England region (Chetty, Hendren, Kline, Saez, & Turner, 2014). To better understand underlying causes of these geographic differences, the diversity of industry and shifts in the work landscape may contribute to these varying outcomes.

In the past few decades, the US has experienced a period of "deindustrialization" marked by closing factories and declining manufacturing jobs. Furthermore, industries based on natural resources (e.g. mining) have decreased, and along with these industries, so too has the median income in rural communities dropped (Monnat, 2016). While the economic crisis is not exclusive to rural communities since small working-class cities built on manufacturing are also suffering, health in rural America is deteriorating. Life expectancy is declining and rates of drug and alcohol abuse, suicides, and obesity are increasing (Monnat & Brown, 2018). Research has demonstrated a relationship between county-level economic distress (i.e. poverty, unemployment, economic inequality) and drug-related mortalities (Monnat, 2018). In the same study, results have shown that counties with labor markets reliant on mining were correlated with these fatalities, whereas those dependent on government sector jobs were associated with lower rates, perhaps due to their stability and lower levels of physical stress. Similarly, interview data from individuals who accidentally overdosed on opioids in a Pennsylvania community based on manufacturing, revealed associations between these instances and feelings of hopelessness amid a bleak labor market (McLean, 2016).

Whereas diminishing industries may be replaced with burgeoning technology industries in urban centers and opportunities for further training and education are abundant, fewer opportunities exist to fill a similar void in more isolated communities; moreover, mental health and medical services are scarcer to support suffering individuals when needed (Monnat, 2016). If working-class individuals can find work, escaping from the increasing economic divide in the US may prove insurmountable considering that those with college degrees earn 70% more than their peers with solely high school diplomas (Corak, 2013). Comparatively, a college degree is associated with 30% higher income in Canada. These statistics highlight the barriers to intergenerational mobility in poor and working-class communities and these barriers are compounded for people of color. While popular media portrayed rural communities as almost entirely White following the 2016 Presidential election, these regions consist of 20% of people of color

(Monnat & Brown, 2018). Taken together, the information put forth suggests an eroding

environment for many US citizens, marked by mental illness and drug related-fatalities

tied to job loss and hopelessness. The plight of individuals in rural and working-class

communities has been an emphasis of the preceding section to exemplify cases in which

bleak opportunities, and associated consequences, for individuals with low SES

backgrounds may be exacerbated in communities with declining work opportunities.

However, these realities point to the need to incorporate geographic and social-class

related factors, beyond rural areas, in research to better understand complex associations

among unemployment, work volition, access to decent work, and mental health. Thus, the

present study sought to integrate community level economic inequality and

unemployment rates when exploring these relationships.

Economic Hardship and Inequality

The previous sections on economic collapse and areas with depleted industries

reveal devastating consequences of economic hardship. While SES is a well-established

social determinant of health (Solar & Irwin, 2018), some scholars posit that "measures of

relative deprivation" may mediate the relationship between SES and well-being (Diemer

et al., 2013). Accordingly, economic and psychological researchers have revealed

economic inequality, as opposed to absolute poverty, as a stronger predictor of mental

and physical health in societies (Fine et al., 2010), and neighborhoods with greater

upward mobility are associated with lower levels of economic inequality (Chetty, &

Hendren, 2018). Numerous theories from sociology, social psychology, and public

health, among others, advance theories for explaining deleterious effects of inequality, including its impact on access to resources, disruption of community cohesion, and individual perceptions (e.g. work volition) (Fine et al., 2010; Kawachi, Kennedy, & Glass, 1999; Patel, 2018; Putnam, 2000). Accordingly, these theories appear interspersed throughout the review to help explain empirical findings as they are presented.

In a meta-analysis of 26 studies in high-income countries, economic inequality was positively associated with high rates of depression (Patel, 2018). At this national-level of analysis, researchers used the neo-material hypothesis to explain these differences. Namely, countries with a smaller income gap are associated with greater provision of social services to its citizens (Patel, 2018), thus attenuating the development of mental health issues. Along with this level of analysis, researchers (e.g., Kennedy, Kawachi, Glass, & Prothrow-Stith, 1998) have called for further exploration on neighborhood and individual levels to better understand how income inequality relates to an individual's psychological experience and interactions with others.

Narrowing in on a US context, researchers investigated the impact of economic inequality on well-being by classifying states according to varying degrees of economic inequality using the Gini coefficient, a statistical measure of wealth distribution in a given geographic region, and correlating these categories with individual self-reports of health in a multilevel analysis (Kennedy et al., 1998). To measure health, researchers utilized one survey item asking respondents to rate their general health according to a Likert scale (poor, fair, good, very good) and then dichotomized the variable. Results indicated that poorer health was associated with greater state-level inequality. While the study contributes to our understanding of economic inequality's impact on general health in the US, it fails to capture its relationship to mental health and to account for substantial within-state differences. To this end, Monnat (2018) explored associations between county-level variables and drug-related mortality rates. Findings revealed disparities in death rates according to county-level economic stress, an index encompassing poverty, unemployment, and secondary education rates, and economic inequality (Gini coefficient), with greater economic stress correlated with higher mortality rates. Additional research at the county-level, targeting elderly adults, revealed a relationship between income inequality rates and reports of depression (Muramotsa, 2003). Notably, this relationship persisted even after controlling for individual SES, suggesting that community inequality contributes unique variance to health outcomes above and beyond SES. Although these findings highlight the critical role of community inequality in the established relationship between economic constraints and mental health work, moderation analyses may prove fruitful in exposing variations to these patterns.

Several theories have attempted to explain the grave impact of economic inequality on well-being. For instance, social comparison theory maintains that people tend to compare themselves with others when assessing their social position, and that negative appraisals of wealth and status in comparison to others cause psychological distress (Festinger, 1954; Fine et al., 2010; Kawachi et al., 1998). An extant study found support for this theory in that county income inequality moderated the association of relative income (perception of income in comparison to others) with life satisfaction, as measured by a single indicator assessing a person's satisfaction with their life (Cheung & Lucas, 2016). As predicted, researchers found a negative association between relative income and life satisfaction. Furthermore, the relationship was more pronounced in counties with high Gini coefficients and for low-income people, highlighting the need to attend to group differences in future research.

Much of the extant research on the effects of income inequality employs the Gini coefficient as a measure. While the Gini coefficient can provide a large-scale view of inequality, such as in national comparisons, the coefficient is less stable at a county level as it is sensitive to outliers and one extremely wealthy individual may pull the coefficient upward. For smaller units of analysis (e.g. counties), other measures of inequality are therefore recommended, such as various ratios or the percentage of people earning over a certain annual income (Zimmerman & Bell, 2006). For instance, in a study of county-level income inequality and mortality rates, researchers utilized a 90/10 ratio for inequality: that is, the percent of individuals in the 90th income percentile compared to the percent of those in the 10th percentile (McLaughlin& Stokes, 2002). In addition to producing further support for the negative impact of economic inequality, the study explored the moderating impact of race. Interestingly, researchers found a negative relationship between economic inequality and mortality rates for Black people. While this finding may appear counterintuitive, researchers hypothesized that when Black people reside in low inequality communities, it may be associated with a higher concentration of Black people, which have historically been underserved. This study highlights the importance of exploring how different groups of people, particularly those from historically marginalized backgrounds, experience economic conditions at a community level and how these experiences may exacerbate or inhibit various health outcomes. Furthermore, some research has documented associations of both higher levels of racial segregation and economic inequality, with lower levels of upward mobility (Chetty,

Hendren, & Katz, 2016), thus warranting further investigation to clarify the complex relationships among health, access to decent work, and economic inequality.

Thus far, this review of the literature has demonstrated the powerful role of economic inequality on mental and physical health from reports of general health and life satisfaction to depression and mortality rates, including fatal deaths from suicide and opioid overdoses. Increasing inequality rates are byproducts of larger economic and political shifts, hitting communities with declining industries and limited economic resources the hardest, often found in rural areas and outside of major urban centers. Given the impact of changing labor markets on access to decent work and the role of decent work on well-being, further research is needed to understand the role of community economic inequality in access to decent work. Because social comparison theory (Festinger, 1954) involves perceptions of one's social position, it follows that income inequality may impact attainment of decent work by disrupting the relationship between economic constraints and work volition, also a perception. Put another way, inequality may inhibit the path to work volition, in turn, limiting access to decent work and further exacerbating the relationship between inequality and decent work.

As reflected in the material reviewed thus far, literature on economic inequality has shown how a community-level economic factor can impact individual outcomes related to upward mobility and mental and physical health. Similarly, research on county-level unemployment rates suggests a related phenomenon by which community factors influence individuals (Helliwell & Huang, 2014). Corroborating results on links between work and well-being (Paul & Moser, 2009; Swanson, 2012), researchers have demonstrated that unemployment was negatively correlated with subjective well-being.

Perhaps more novel in its contribution, Helliwell and Huang revealed that unemployment rates had a stronger significant indirect impact of employed individuals, such that higher county-level unemployment rates were more strongly associated with poorer subjective well-being in employed people than the unemployed. Researchers speculated that higher unemployment rates may cause those with jobs to anticipate further job loss in a community and therefore their own job loss (Helliwell & Huang, 2014). Applying this reasoning to work volition, it follows that people's perceptions of choice in work opportunities may decline. Related to social capital theories, Helliwell and Huang (2014) also hypothesized that people may interpret increasing unemployment rates as an indicator of increasing social disorganization, and anticipate other negative consequences along with unemployment, such as increasing crime rates.

Given the breadth of literature on the harmful impact of community economic inequality, unemployment rates, and economic conditions more broadly, the present study explored potential moderation effects of economic conditions in relationships between social class and work volition, as well as social class and well-being. To measure economic conditions, the study will employ measures of economic inequality, unemployment rates, and median income. The 80/20 ratio will be used for economic inequality because economists have suggested that this is a more robust indicator of inequality that individuals might encounter on a daily basis (Zimmerman & Bell, 2006). The 80/20 ratio represents the difference in income between the household at the 80th percentile of income and the household at the 20th percentile. The ratio thus provides a picture of the disparity of the wealthiest fifth of households in comparison to households in the poorest. The unemployment rate captures the number of individuals searching and available to work, in comparison to the number of people who are active in the labor force and those who are unemployed (BLS, 2018). The median income will be used because it represents a more stable marker of community income in comparison to a mean which is susceptible to being skewed by outliers (Opportunity Nation & Measure of America, 2017). Integrating county-level economic conditions into explorations of individual-level relationships among social class, work volition, access to decent work and well-being, thus offers a unique contribution to our understanding of work experiences in the US through a PWF/PWT perspective (Blustein, 2006; Duffy et al., 2016).

Social capital

Situated in social comparison theory (Festinger, 1954), the previous sections shed light on how work volition and life satisfaction may be impacted by negative evaluations of one's self and opportunities for decent work, driven by economic conditions, such as unemployment rates and economic inequality. The analysis thus far has introduced the impact of economic capital by examining various dimensions of economic conditions and has begun to investigate how these dimensions relate to individuals' psychological experience in relation to one another, as well as how economic conditions may disrupt access to other resources and opportunity, such as social capital. The following sections will more fully explicate these recursive relationships among economic conditions and social capital, by providing additional social capital theoretical background and conceptualizing other forms of community opportunity, such as community engagement and education, as social capital, in addition to representing overlapping domains of economic conditions, to better understand access and attainment of decent work.

Research has demonstrated associations between the community where children grow up and their income in adulthood (Chetty & Hendren, 2016). Chetty and Hendren (2016) hypothesize that high opportunity areas are less segregated by income and therefore children have greater access to social capital (SC), often conceptualized as the networks of relationships (structural) and cohesiveness of a community consisting of these networks (Putnam, 2000). The social networks to which an individual belongs and contributes may include relationships with family, friends and neighbors, membership in community organizations and civic engagement, such as volunteering and voting. Relatedly, cognitive SC describes perceptions of social cohesion, trust, reciprocity, and shared norms. (Kawachi et al., 1999). SC may serve a protective function by expanding networks that can be relied upon for emotional and instrumental support in times of need. For instance, research has highlighted the value of social capital as a major component of community resilience in the wake of natural disasters (Aldrich & Meyer, 2015). Consistent with this hypothesis, extant literature has demonstrated associations between social capital and positive mental health outcomes. SC at a county-level, measured by concentration of civic organizations, voting, census response rate, tax-exempt non-profits, was strongly negatively associated with opioid drug overdoses (Zoorob & Salemi, 2017). Furthermore, Monnat (2018) showed that economic factors alone cannot account for disparities in drug-related mortalities because religious organizations were associated with lower death rates. Based on these findings, SC may buffer against the negative impact of unemployment which might be considered a collective trauma or loss (Abramovitz & Albrecht, 2013).

Along with disrupting access to SC through income segregation (Chetty & Hendren, 2016), economic inequality may disrupt SC in communities by instigating distrust, garnering skepticism regarding fairness (Wilmot & Dauner, 2017); relatedly, perceptions of relative deprivation may foster feelings of shame and lead to social withdrawal. Accordingly, withdrawal may inhibit people from accessing SC, and decrease sources of social support, which PWT posits plays a protective role for marginalized individuals attempting to access decent work (Duffy et al., 2016). These processes not only hurt the individual but the community at large according to Putnam (2000), who maintains that utilizing one's social connections creates benefit to the community. Accordingly, even individuals with limited economic resources may benefit from social capital at a community level. Relatedly, studies have demonstrated interdependent relationships between economic hardship and community involvement. For instance, researchers found that both unemployment rates and state level economic inequality were negatively correlated with civic engagement, along with greater civic participation observed among those employed in comparison to those who were not employed (Lim & Sander, 2013). Lim and Sander (2013) hypothesized that although civic engagement, such as volunteering, has the potential to foster the development of new skills among those unemployed and to positively impact self-esteem, unemployment rates may conflict with these results by decreasing motivation in a climate that may appear unfair and take a backseat to focusing on obtaining work to meet important survival needs.

Findings thus far illustrate multifaceted effects of community economic conditions, such as the potential to undermine formation of work volition, which is positively correlated with decent work, as well as by impeding the development of beneficial social resources, such as social support and civic engagement, both of which benefit individuals and their community. Therefore, the present study will incorporate a global community opportunity index, which incorporates several indicators of community and civic engagement, such as the rate of disconnected youth, the rate of individuals 16 to 24 who are neither working nor in school (Opportunity Nation & Measure of America, 2017), to better understand how community engagement impacts the relationships between social class and work volition, and between social class and life satisfaction, according to the PWT model. Research has demonstrated that rates of disconnected youth serve as the greatest predictor of overall opportunity at a state level and as the second greatest predictor at the county level (Opportunity Nation & Measure of America, 2017). Furthermore, this age group faces a critical time period in the transition from school-to-work; a breadth of research has focused on the importance career development process and interventions with this age range (Ali et al., 2013; Perry & Wallace). Thus, the percent of disconnected youth in a community is likely indicative of resources and supports available to this age group, and it follows that these resources may be a marker for the overall landscape in which all adults are able to access decent work.

Education. The previous section detailed relationships among economic conditions and community engagement through a social capital lens, with community involvement serving as both a form and outcome of social capital that is implicated in community economic conditions. Considering the integral role of educational opportunities in access to decent work and upward mobility (Chetty & Hendren, 2016), the present study would be remiss not to incorporate community education opportunity in its design, particularly given its focus on social class. Consistent with social capital theory (Putnam, 2000), education forums serve as a structure in which social networks form, with higher education facilities and schools in more affluent neighborhoods, conferring greater prestige and with this prestige, greater access to opportunities through connections and accruement of cultural capital (Lareau, 2011). Exemplifying this principle, data from a quasi-experiment (Moving to Opportunity) revealed that college attendance rates were significantly greater for individuals whose families moved to neighborhoods with lower levels of poverty when they were children in comparison to individuals whose families did not (Chetty et al., 2016). Furthermore, education attainment has been correlated with greater income, better health, and lifetime satisfaction (Child Trends DataBank, 2016). Thus, research suggests the intertwined nature of economic conditions and education, as well as the role of community education opportunities in several important work-related and well-being outcomes. To capture this important element, the present study utilizes county-level rates of pre-kindergarten enrollment, on-time high school graduation, and percent of people with Associates degrees or higher, as indicators of community educational opportunity. Research has demonstrated that rates of people with Associates degrees and higher is the greatest predictor of overall community opportunity (Opportunity Nation & Measure of America, 2017).

Present Study

Amid economic and social upheaval, public health, political, and economic researchers have begun to examine manifestations of increasing inequality, job loss, and changing labor markets on access to decent work and well-being. In response to

MacLachan's charge (2014), counseling psychology can integrate these macrolevel factors with individual psychological variables to better understand individuals' experiences in traditionally neglected populations, such as those in predominantly working-class communities. With this spirit, the present study integrated community and individual factors in an attempt to investigate specific pathways by which individual economic constraints impact work and work-related variables, as well as mental health, and the role of community economic conditions and opportunity. To achieve this aim, I used structural equation modeling (SEM) analyses to test the following hypotheses.

Hypotheses

1. Prior research on social class and work-related outcomes has demonstrated that lower social class background is associated with lower levels of career aspirations, outcome expectations, self-efficacy in career decision-making, and value in occupational prestige (Brown et al., 1996; Metheny & McWhirter, 2013; Perry & Wallace, 2013; Thompson & Dahling, 2010). Furthermore, individuals from poor and working-class backgrounds must put their survival needs first, often at the expense of pursuing careers that may be more interesting and intrinsically motivating (Blustein, 2006; Shah, Mullainathan, & Shafir, 2012). Taken together, these findings suggest that people from lower class backgrounds are often limited in their work choices and accessing decent work, which in turn impacts overall life satisfaction. Thus, I hypothesize that:

   a. Social class will be positively associated with the outcomes of life satisfaction, decent work, and work volition. Namely, higher social class will be associated with greater levels of these three variables.

2. Several researchers have demonstrated associations between work volition and positive work-related outcomes (Duffy et al., 2012). Initial studies utilizing the PWT model have demonstrated that work volition mediates the association between social class and decent work, and that work volition positively predicts access to decent work (Douglass et al., 2017; Duffy et al., 2016; Duffy et al., 2019). Therefore, consistent with previous findings, I hypothesize that:

   a. Work volition will be positively associated with decent work.

   b. Work volition will mediate the positive relationship from social class to decent work.

3. Fewer studies have tested hypothesized links between decent work and variables related to well-being, such as life satisfaction, in the PWT model. A couple of studies have demonstrated a positive direct association (Kozan et al., 2019) and positive indirect association through the mediator of needs satisfaction (Duffy, Kim et al., 2019). While the present model does not include PWT needs as a mediator, I hypothesize that:

   a. Decent work will be positively associated with life satisfaction.

4. Research has demonstrated that economic hardship, such as poverty, unemployment, and economic inequality, has detrimental impacts on physical and mental health, as well as on social mobility (Cheng & Lucas, 2016; Monnat, 2016; Muramotsa, 2003). Scholars have used social capital, social comparison, and relative deprivation theories to explain how inequality can impact individual perceptions through negative appraisals of one's self and their opportunities. Accordingly, I hypothesize that:

a. Community economic conditions and opportunity will moderate the
    relationship between social class and work volition.

b. Community economic conditions and opportunity will moderate the
    pathway from social class to life satisfaction.

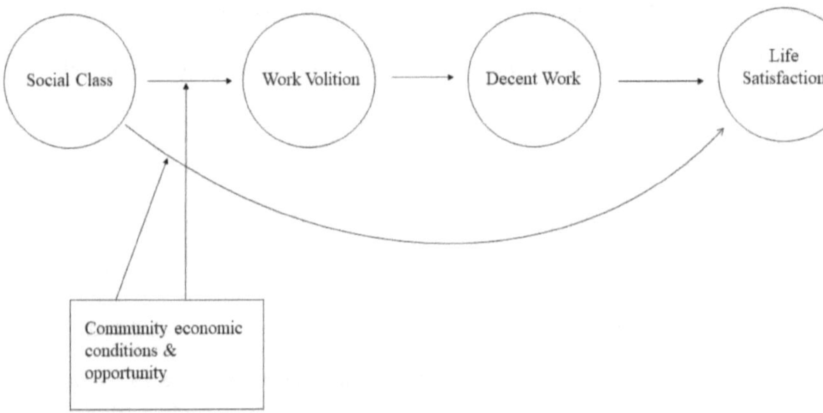

Figure 1. Hypothesized full structural model

Chapter 3

Methods

Design

The current cross-sectional study relied on a descriptive, quantitative design, utilizing structural equation modeling (SEM). SEM allows for examination of latent variables through measurement models, as well as structural models to test hypothesized direct and indirect pathways and overall model fit. Scholars suggest using SEM when testing for complex mediation and moderation models (Baron & Kenny, 1986; Fassinger, 1987; Martens, 2005). I used RStudio for running measurement and structural equation models. Prior to running preliminary analyses, I geocoded the data by merging individual-level data with county-level from secondary datasets (e.g. Bureau of Labor Statistics, US Census, etc.) by matching participant IP addresses to county-level, Federal Information Processing Standard (FIPS) codes. The dataset used in this study was derived from a larger scale quantitative project that has been exploring the relationship between conditions of work and related predictors and outcomes (Blustein et al., under review). However, the present study is unique in its focus on social class and an economic conditions moderator, and it relies on modeling PWT-derived hypotheses that are not covered in the other studies.

Participants

The sample consisted of 816 US adult participants with a mean age of 35.7 years (SD=10.23). This sample size meets criteria for power of 0.85 according to Jackson's (2003) guidelines for latent SEM models. Participants self-identified their gender as man (*n*= 503, 61.6 %), woman (*n*=307, 37.6%), Transgender (*n*=1, 0.1 %), and other (*n*=5, 0.6%). According to self-report, participants identified their race/ethnicity as African American (*n*=101, 12.4%), Native American (*n*=15, 1.8%), Arab American (*n*=1, 0.1%), Asian American (*n*=50, 6.1%), South Asian (*n*=7, 0.9%), Latinx (*n*=48, 5.9%), Pacific Islander (*n*=1, 0.1%), European American (*n*=624, 76.5%), and Other (*n*=5, 0.6%). In terms of employment, 498 (61.0%) participants endorsed that they would be employed within the next 12 months, 224 (27.5%) were unsure and 97 (11.9%) disagreed. Eight (1.0%) participants reported their highest degree as less than a high school degree, 89 as a high school degree (10.9%), 38 as trade/vocational school (4.7%), 187 as some college (22.9%), 409 as a college degree (50.1%), and 84 as a graduate degree (10.3%). Of note, 60.4% of the sample reported holding a bachelor's degree or higher, which is substantially higher than the general population, which is approximately 36.0% according to 2019 US Census Bureau data. According to self-report, the sample's class breakdown was lower class (*n* = 58, 7.1%), working class (*n* = 286, 35.0%), middle class (*n* = 385, 47.2%), upper middle class (*n* = 80, 9.8%), and upper class (*n* = 1, 0.1%).

Measures

All measures are presented in Appendix B.

Demographic characteristics. Participants completed a demographic section within the survey that contained questions about gender, age, sexual orientation, ethnic/racial identity, highest educational degree obtained and employment security.

Social Class. Social class was measured by three indicators reviewed next: annual median income (objective social class) childhood social class (subjective social class), and current social class (based on self-report.

Table 1

Demographic Characteristics for Sample (n=816)

Participant Variables		n	Percentage
Gender			
	Man	503	61.4
	Woman	307	37.6
	Transgender	1	0.1
	Other	5	0.6
Race/ethnicity			
	African American	101	12.4
	Native American	15	1.8
	Arab American	1	0.1
	Asian American	50	6.1
	South Asian	7	0.9
	Latinx	48	5.9
	Pacific Islander	1	0.1
	European American	694	76.5
	Other	5	0.6
Highest Level of Education			
	Less Than High School	8	1.0
	High School Degree	89	10.9
	Trade/Vocational School	38	4.7
	Some College	187	22.9
	College Degree	409	50.1
	Graduate Degree	84	10.3

Objective Social Class. Objective social class was measured by annual median

income and was assessed by asking participants, "What is your average yearly income?"

and they were given 10 forced choice options, including *1*=Less than $25,000 per year,

2=$25,000-$50,000 per year, *3*=$51,000-$75,000 per year..., *9*=$201,000 + per year and

an option indicating "I don't know". This question and all 10 responses is presented in

Appendix B. Yearly income is a commonly used indicator of objective SES in social science research (Diemer et al., 2013).

Subjective Social Class. Subjective social class was assessed by two indicator variables – *childhood social class* and *current social class.*

Childhood Social Class. Participants responded to a single forced-choice question asking, "How would you identify your childhood social class?" and chose from the following options, *1*=Lower class, *2*=Working class, *3*=Middle class, *4*=Upper middle class, *5*=Upper class. Perceptions of social class is a commonly used indicator of subjective social class in social science research (Liu et al., 2004).

Current Social Class. Similarly, Participants responded to a single forced-choice question asking, "How would you identify your social class?" and chose from the same five options, *1*=Lower class, *2*=Working class, *3*=Middle class, *4*=Upper middle class, *5*=Upper class.

Work Volition. The 4-item Volition subscale from the Work Volition Scale (WVS; Duffy, Diemer et al., 2012b) was used to assess levels of work volition. The brief measure employs a 7-point Likert-type scale ranging from strongly disagree to strongly agree, with higher scores representing greater perceptions of volition. An example scale item includes, "I feel total control over my job choices.'' Duffy, Diemer et al. (2012) produced an internal consistency of $\alpha =. 78$, and additional studies have demonstrated strong internal consistency and stable relationships to related constructs, such as barriers and sense of control (e.g., Douglas et al., 2017; Kim et al., 2020).

Decent work. The Decent Work Scale (DWS; Duffy et al., 2017) assesses five components of decent work: safe working conditions, adequate compensation, access to healthcare, adequate rest and free time, and a match of organizational and social/family values. Participants responded to items on a seven-point Likert scale ranging from *Strongly disagree* to *Strongly agree.* Example items include, "I feel emotionally safe interacting with people at work" and "I have free time during the work week." Research has demonstrated excellent internal consistency ($\propto$ = .91; Duffy et al., 2017; Douglass et al., 2017; Duffy et al., 2018). Researchers recommend testing the DWS as a bifactor model, including one global decent work score totaled from all 15 items and as five unique scores representing the five components of decent work by totaling the three items associated with each subscale (Duffy et al., 2017; Duffy et al. 2018). Higher scores on both the global factor and five subfactors indicate greater decent work and lower scores represent less decent work. Research has demonstrated strong predictive validity as decent work correlated with job satisfaction, work meaning, and withdrawal intentions (Duffy et al., 2017). Cronbach's alpha in the current study was 0.9 for the global scale and as follows for each component: safe ($\propto$ = 0.84), health ($\propto$ = 0.97), compensation ($\propto$ = 0.85), rest ($\propto$ = 0.80), and values ($\propto$ = 0.94).

Life Satisfaction. The Satisfaction with Life Scale (SWLS; Diener, Emmons, Larson & Griffin, 1985) is a 5-item measure using a 7-point Likert scale that ranges from 1 (strongly disagree) to 7 (strongly agree). Sample items include, "In most ways, my life is close to my ideal" and "If I could live my life over, I would change almost nothing." This widely cited scale has demonstrated high internal consistency in research (Pavot, Diener, & Diener, 2009) and α =.91 in a recent study (Autin et al., 2019). A total score will be computed by adding all items, with higher scores representing greater satisfaction with life and lower scores representing lower levels of satisfaction with life.

The scale has been used widely and demonstrated excellent psychometric properties. Cronbach's alpha for the current study was 0.93.

Moderator Variables: Moderator variables include a global Community Opportunity index, a global Economic Conditions index, and several indicators of the Economic Conditions index.

Community Economic Conditions. A composite score comprised of the indicators of county-level unemployment rates, median income, poverty rates, and an 80/20 ratio of economic inequality will measure community economic conditions.

Unemployment rates. Local unemployment statistics from the Bureau of Labor Statistics (BLS) report unemployment rates as the percentage of individuals actively seeking and available to work in the preceding four-week period in comparison to the total labor force (BLS). Rates used in calculating the economic opportunity composite score are from 2017.

Median household income. County median household is the midpoint income when all household incomes are arranged from the highest to lowest in the county. Sources of income may include earnings from employment, interest, pensions, social security benefits, and unemployment, among others. The mean income of a county is much higher than the median because income is not evenly distributed and thus median income serves as a more representative measure of a typical household income (Opportunity Nation & Measure of America, 2019). County-level median household income data is provided by the U.S. Census Bureau, American Community Survey and were collected from 2011-2015.

Poverty rates. The county poverty rate is the percentage of people living below the federal poverty rate in comparison the total number of people living in the county. County-level poverty rates are provided by the U.S. Census Bureau, American Community Survey and were collected from 2011-2015.

80/20 ratio. The 80/20 ratio represents the difference in income between household income at the 80th percentile and the household income at the 20th percentile. The ratio thus provides a picture of the disparity of the wealthiest fifth of households in comparison to households in the poorest fifth. Opportunity Nation and Measure of America (2017) calculated this ratio for counties using income data provided by the U.S. Census Bureau, American Community Survey and were collected from 2011-2015.

Prior to computing a total composite score, indicators will be rescaled to enable comparisons. The highest and lowest scores on observed variables will be compared the highest and lowest possible scores according to the following formula:

$$\text{Observed value rescaled} = \frac{(\text{Observed value} - \text{Lowest value})}{\text{Highest value} - \text{Lowest value}} \times 100$$

Variables vary in their directionality. For instance, higher poverty rates represent less economic opportunity whereas higher median income represents greater economic opportunity. To allow for comparisons, all indicators that are negative in their directionality will be rescaled to have positive directionality, using the following formula:

$$\text{Observed value rescaled} = 1 - \frac{(\text{Observed value} - \text{Lowest value})}{\text{Highest value} - \text{Lowest value}} \times 100$$

The composite economic opportunity score will be computed by averaging the four standardized variables and will range from 0 to 100, with higher scores representing greater opportunity and lower scores indicating less opportunity.

Community Opportunity. A composite score comprised of four indices – Economic Conditions, Education, Health, and Community (e.g. civic engagement) – will measure overall community opportunity. The four indices each consist of several indicators, and the 17 indicators constitute overall community opportunity. Indicators for the aforementioned Economic Conditions index are described above. Data collected between 2011 and 2015 from the U.S. Census Bureau, American Community Survey provided most of the indicators for the other three indices, such as pre-school enrollment for the Education index, health insurance for the Health index and voter registration for the Community index. Additional sources of data include the Bureau of Health Workforce, the Bureau of CDC, and Bureau of Justice Statistics, among others. Opportunity Nation and Measure of America (2019) collated the data and calculated the indicators, four index scores, and overall Community Opportunity index. A full list of the 17 indicators, along with their data sources and calculations are presented in Appendix B.

Chapter 4

Results

Overview of Analyses

This chapter presents results from preliminary and primary study analyses. Following a description of preliminary analyses, the process of specifying measurement models to establish latent structures for the major study variables through confirmatory factor analyses is detailed. Two measurement models are described before presenting model fit indices for two full SEM models with varying latent construct structures for decent work. The next section describes estimation and significance testing of mediation pathways from social class to decent work via the mediator of work volition in each SEM model. After establishing the direct and indirect relations in the full models, moderation analyses are presented. Several measures of economic conditions and other community opportunity indices were tested as moderators in regression analyses with manifest variables from social class to work volition, and from social class to life satisfaction. These moderation analyses were conducted using interaction terms between social class and moderating variables., All analyses were conducted in Version 1.2.503 of Rstudio, and unless otherwise specified, using Version 6.3.6 of base R (R Core Team, 2020).

Preliminary Analyses

Prior to running analyses to test the study's major hypotheses, I examined missing data and explored the distribution of data for normality before running bivariate correlations of the study's primary manifest variables. These correlations are presented in

Table 3. The psych package was used to compute descriptive statistics and correlations (Revelle, 2019).

Missing data. After deleting cases based on the data screening procedures outlined above, I analyzed missingness at the item level and determined the data to be missing at random (MAR). I addressed the missing values using multiple imputation, which pools estimates from five imputed data sets (Rubin, 1987). Given the small amount of missing data, multiple imputation should not produce significantly different results from alternate missing data techniques, such as full-information maximum likelihood (FMIL) (Allison, 2003; Widaman, 2006). The mice (Multivariate Imputation by Chained Equations) (van Buuren & Groothuis-Oudshoorn, 2011), semTools (Jorgensen et al., 2019) and lavaan packages (Rosseel, 2012) were used in combination to impute missing data.

Distribution of variables. Descriptive statistics for major study variables, including means, standard deviations, and statistics for skewness and kurtosis are reported in Table 2. The distribution of data was assessed for normality, including for skewness and kurtosis, by checking descriptive statistics for outliers and visually inspecting histograms of major study variables. Variables appear to have met criteria for univariate normality, given that standard errors for skewness and kurtosis were within +/- 2 and +/-3, respectively, and histograms appeared normally distributed.

Primary Analyses

Latent structural equation modeling comprised the study's primary analyses. Before testing the measurement model representing the latent constructs to ensure the fundamental elements of the structural model produced adequate fit, confirmatory factor analysis explored the fit of varying Decent Work (DW) structures. After testing the fit of two possible measurement models, I specified two structural models according to hypothesized direct and indirect pathways. To assess these models, I utilized three fit indices – the Comparative Fit Index (CFI), the Tucker-Lewis Index and the root mean-square error of approximation (RMSEA). The CFI and TLI are incremental fit indices, meaning they compare the specified model to the baseline or null model. CFI/TLI statistics ≥ 0.95 are typically considered good fit and ≥ 0.90 are acceptable (West & Gore, 2006).The RMSEA statistic is an absolute fit index and is sensitive to model mis-specification, which means that the specified model is compared to the best possible fitting model for the data and RMSEA <.08 is reasonable fit and <.05 is close fit (Kline, 2015; McDonald & Ho, 2002). Although chi-square ($\chi2$) is another index of inadequate fit, it is oversensitive in moderate to large samples (Tabachnick & Fidell, 2013). Given the current sample size, the chi-square ($\chi2$) may not provide an accurate estimate of fit. The modeling analyses were conducted using robust maximum likelihood (MLR) estimation of huber white standard errors to account for possible deviations in normality of the data. CFA and SEM analyses were conducted using the lavaan package (Rosseel, 2012).

Measurement Models

The hypothesized measurement model contained the following latent variables: social class, work volition, decent work and life satisfaction. Prior to constructing the measurement model, I conducted confirmatory factor analysis (CFA) with three proposed latent structures for the Decent Work construct (Duffy et al., 2017).

Table 2

Descriptive Statistics of Measured Variables (n=816)

Variable	Scale Mean	SD	Min	Max	Skewness	Kurtosis
Income	2.9	1.55	1	10	1.4	2.42
Child SC	2.61	0.91	1	5	-0.06	-0.41
SC	2.60	0.77	1	5	-0.13	-0.25
Volition	4.66	1.48	1	7	-0.53	-0.39
Decent Work	4.83	1.16	1	7	-0.53	-.08
Safe	5.82	1.15	1	7	-1.36	2.2
Health	4.54	2.07	1	7	-0.55	-1.08
Compensation	4.33	1.7	1	7	-0.12	-0.97
Rest	4.66	1.58	1	7	-0.29	-0.83
Values	4.81	1.55	1	7	-0.63	-0.19
Life Satisfaction	4.51	1.66	1	6	-.48	-.8

Table 3

Correlation Matrix of Measured Manifest Variables (n=816)

Measure	1	2	3	4	5	6	7	8	9	10	11
1. Income	-										
2. Child class	.16**	-									
3. Class	.39**	.58**	-								
4. Volition	.25**	.16**	.39**	-							
5. DW	.24**	.14**	.34**	.61**	-						
6. Safe	.10**	.11**	.16**	.40**	.64**	-					
7. Health	.31**	.15**	.41**	.46**	.73**	.29**	-				
8. Comp	.17	.07*	.22**	.42**	.78**	.34**	.45**	-			
9. Rest	.05**	.05*	.08*	.36**	.67**	.41**	.21**	.49**	-		
10. Values	.17**	.13**	.29**	.56**	.77**	.48**	.48**	.47**	.38**	-	
11. Life Sat	.25**	.10**	.33**	.49**	.41**	.25**	.32**	.33**	.20**	0.38**	-

Note: ** *p* < .01. * *p*<.05

Confirmatory factor analyses. Scale developers propose three possible latent factor structures for assessing decent work and recommend using a bifactor approach when possible (Duffy et al., 2017). Consistent with this recommendation, I first conducted a CFA with all 15 items from the Decent Work Scale (DWS) loading onto one global factor and three of the 15 items loading onto each of the five sub-factors (i.e. safe condition, access to healthcare, rest/time off, values), creating six latent factors in the model. Within this structure, I did not allow any factors to correlate by constraining the covariances to zero. The bifactor model produced acceptable fit to the data: χ^2 (75) = 342.60, $p < .001$, TLI = 1.00, CFI = .96, and RMSEA = .08, 90% CI [0.075, 0.093] and factor loadings for all variables ranged from.31 to .88. Factor loadings are presented in Figure 2.

For exploratory purposes, I also tested the hierarchical and correlational structures. In the hierarchical structure, the five components are specified by their respective three items and the five factors are then loaded onto a global decent work factor as indicators. Some researchers have utilized this approach with promising results (Kozan et al., 2019). In the present study, this structure produced poor fit: χ^2 (85) = 615.16, $p < .001$, TLI = 1.00, CFI = .92, and RMSEA = .11, 90% CI [0.101, 0.117]. The correlational structure consists of five latent factors to represent the five components of decent work, specified again by their respective three item indicators, and the five factors are allowed to correlate in the model. Although the correlational structure produced a better fit than the hierarchical structure, the RMSEA statistic was still somewhat problematic: χ^2 (80) =491.91, $p < .001$, TLI = 1.00, CFI = .94, and RMSEA = .10, 90% CI [0.09, 0.108], and factor loadings for indicators ranged from *.51* to *.96*. Factor loadings and covariances are depicted in Figure 3.

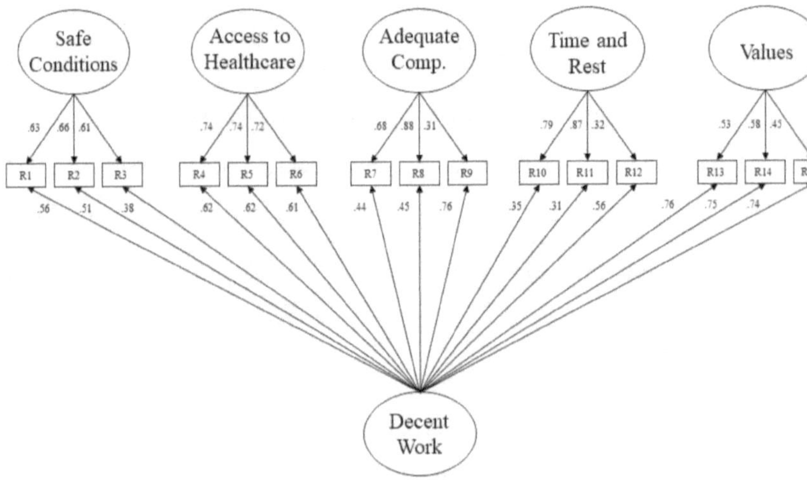

Figure 2. Factor loadings for bifactor model of decent work. Factors were restricted from correlating. All factor loadings are significant at p < .001.

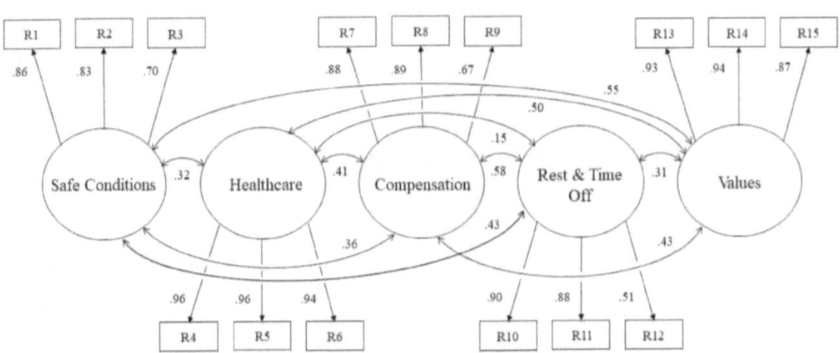

Figure 3. Factor loadings and covariances for correlational model of decent work. All factor loadings and covariances are significant at p < .001.

Overall measurement model. After testing the three structures of decent work, I

assessed the fit of an overall measurement model comprised of the study's major latent variables before conducting structural modeling. Considering the study's aim to explore relationships in the PWT model with the individual subcomponents of DW, I tested the correlational (i.e. five-factor model) structure in the overall measurement model, despite a slightly large RMSEA value. This measurement model produced good fit to the data: χ^2 (296) = 984.86, $p < .001$, TLI = 1.00, CFI = .95, and RMSEA = .06, 90% CI [0.057, 0.066]. Correlations among final latent constructs in this model are reported in Table 4. Using the bifactor structure of DW in the measurement model produced slightly better fit to the data: χ^2 (286) = 751.36, $p < .001$, TLI = 1.00, CFI = .96, and RMSEA = .05, 90% CI [0.047, 0.056]. Both the five-factor and bifactor measurement models were used in separate SEM models in order to examine individual variance from the subcomponents and how this variance changed after accounting for variance from a global factor.

Table 4
Correlations Matrix of Latent Variables (n=816)

Variable	1	2	3	4	5	6	7
1. Social Class	—						
2. Work Volition	.42**	—					
3. Safety	.19**	.48**	—				
4. Healthcare	.42**	.50**	.32**	—			
5. Compensation	.15**	.32**	.32**	.35**	—		
6. Rest/Time	.03**	.28**	.42**	.13**	.61**	—	
7. Values	.30**	.62**	.55**	.50**	.36**	.28**	—
8. Life Satisfaction	.34**	.55**	.30**	.35*	.30**	.16**	.42*

*$p < .05$ **$p < .01$

Structural Modeling

Two models were estimated according to the hypothesized direct pathways with social class predicting work volition, decent work and life satisfaction; work volition predicting decent work; and decent work predicting life satisfaction. While these pathways remained consistent, I tested two versions of the model, utilizing the correlational structure for decent work in the first model and the bi-factor structure in the second. Utilization of the correlational structure allowed for an examination of how the predictors and outcome variables related to the discrete components of decent work. The bifactor structure allowed for an examination of how a global decent work construct functioned in the model, as well as how the discrete components functioned, after controlling for a global factor.

Five-factor structure (correlational)

The full SEM with the factor structure yielded adequate fit: χ^2 (306) = 1362.49, p < .001, TLI = 1.00, CFI = .92, and RMSEA = .075, 90% CI [0.071, 0.079].

Direct relations. As hypothesized, social class significantly predicted work volition and overall life satisfaction. After controlling for work volition to determine the unique direct effect of social class on each of the five components of decent work, social class positively predicted the Healthcare component of decent work. Interestingly, social class appeared to negatively predict the Rest component of decent work. As predicted, work volition was significantly positively associated with all five components of decent work. The Compensation and Values components significantly predicted life satisfaction. Standardized regression coefficients for the significant unique direct effects (p<0.01) are presented in Figure 4. All standardized and unstandardized coefficients are presented in Table A1 in Appendix A.

Indirect relations. Given the results of the direct relations in the full model, work volition appeared to mediate some of the pathways from social class to the various decent work components according to the Baron and Kenny method (1986) for testing mediation. To confirm the potential mediating effects of work volition, I tested regression

coefficients of the indirect pathways. I utilized bootstrapping of standard errors approach

with 500 simulations of the data when specifying indirect paths in the full model

(MacKinnon; Preacher & Hayes, 2004). Monte Carlo confidence intervals (CIs) were

estimated to provide a more precise estimate of indirect effects using the semTools

package (Jorgensen et al., 2019), and effects are significant if zero is not included in the

95% CI. Of note, the CIs were computed on the full dataset (i.e. not with imputed missing

values). Consistent with hypotheses, mediation analyses revealed significant effects for

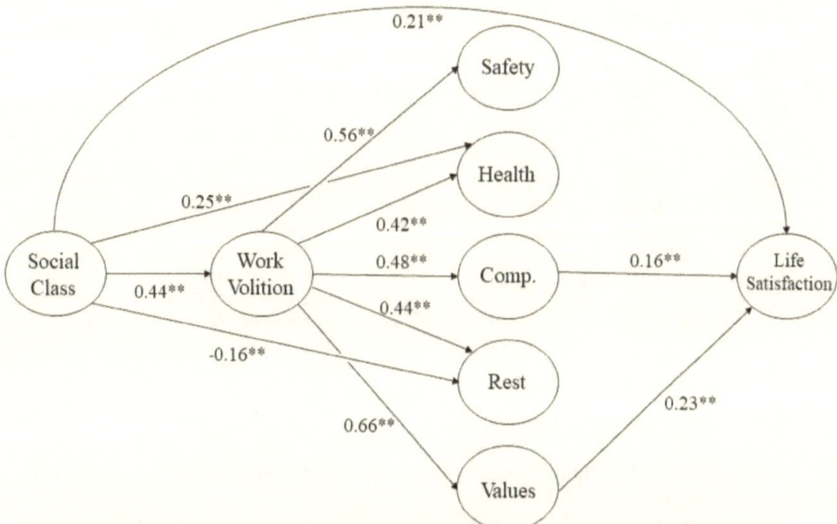

Figure 4. Hypothesized structural model of direct relations between variables using five-factor decent work structure. For parsimony, only significant paths are shown. Values reflect standardized coefficients and are significant at p < .001.

indirect paths specified from social class to each of the five components of decent work through work volition. In comparing direct, indirect and total effects for the five pathways, work volition appears to partially mediate the relationship between social class and the Healthcare and to fully mediate the relationship between social class and the other four components of decent work. Regression coefficients and confidence intervals are presented in Table 5.

Bifactor Structure

Compared to the five-factor model, the bifactor model had good and slightly better fit to the data: χ^2 (351) = 12113.723, $p < .001$, TLI = 1.00, CFI = .96, and RMSEA = .052, 90% CI [0.048, 0.057].

Table 5
Test of Unique Indirect Effects Relations in Five-factor Model (N = 816)

Predictor	Mediator	Outcome	Standardized Indirect Relations	Unstandardized Indirect Relations		95% CI of unstandardized indirect relation	
			β	B	SE	Lower Bound	Upper Bound
Class	Volition	Safety	0.25	0.39	0.07	0.27	0.57
Class	Volition	Health	0.19	0.51	0.08	0.37	0.69
Class	Volition	Comp	0.21	0.48	0.09	0.33	0.77
Class	Volition	Rest	0.19	0.44	0.08	0.31	0.67
Class	Volition	Values	0.29	0.60	0.09	0.44	0.81

Direct relations. As hypothesized, social class significantly positively predicted work volition and Healthcare. Again, social class negatively significantly predicted the Rest component. Contrary to hypotheses, social class did not predict life satisfaction, after accounting for a global decent work variable, and it did not directly predict global DW or the Safety, Compensation and Values components. Work volition positively predicted the global decent work factor but no other DW components. Global DW positively predicted life satisfaction. Standardized regression coefficients for the significant unique direct effects (p<0.01) are presented in Figure 5. All standardized and unstandardized coefficients are presented in Table A2 in Appendix A.

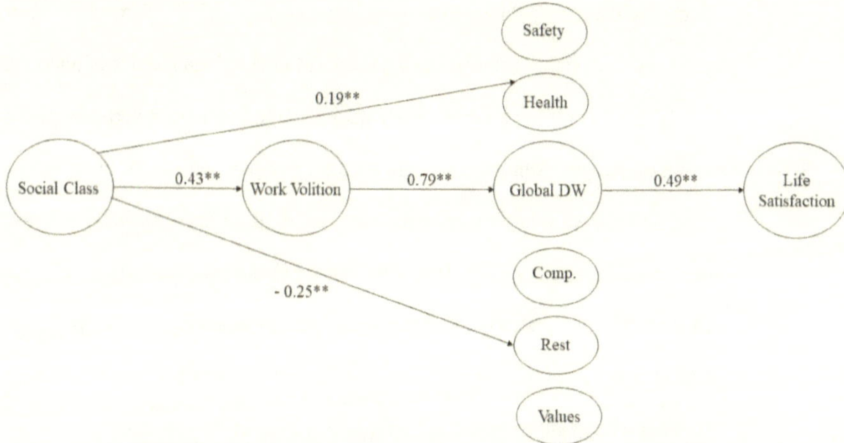

Figure 5. Hypothesized structural model of direct relations between variables using bifactor decent work structure. For parsimony, only significant paths are shown. Values reflect standardized coefficients and are significant at p < .001.

Indirect relations. Although hypotheses predict that social class will indirectly predict all components of decent work and a global DW factor through work volition, results revealed an indirect positive effect on only global DW and indirect negative effects on Healthcare and Values. Regression coefficients and confidence intervals are presented in Table 6. Confidence intervals were computed according to the same aforementioned method as the SEM model with the five-factor construct described above.

Moderation analyses

To determine whether community economic conditions and opportunity impact the hypothesized pathway from social class to work volition and from social class to life satisfaction, I examined several indicators representing these constructs for potential moderating effects. Figure 6 depicts these moderating paths. County-level data comprising the potential economic conditions and community opportunity variables were matched to participants' individual-level data based on their IP addresses. Before specifying moderating pathways in the full SEM model, I ran a series of linear regression models using manifest variables. Moderation analyses with latent variables present several challenges. Although there are several proposed methods for modeling interactions between latent constructs, each carries its limitations and there is not a widely agreed upon approach. Latent Moderated Structural Equations (LMS) method is one approach that is becoming more popular, but unfortunately, it is not possible to conduct in R. Given these limitations, I first sought to determine if an interaction was occurring with manifest variables before pursuing alternate software.

Table 6

Test of Unique Indirect Effects Relations in Bifactor Model (N = 816)

			Standardized Indirect Relations	Unstandardized Indirect Relations		95% CI of unstandardized indirect relation	
Predictor	Mediator	Outcome	β	B	*SE*	Lower Bound	Upper Bound
Class	Volition	Safety	-0.12	-0.16	0.11	-0.38	0.03
Class	Volition	Health	-0.12	-0.25	0.12	-0.49	-0.04
Class	Volition	Comp	-0.32	-0.32	0.27	-0.69	0.12
Class	Volition	Rest	-0.22	-0.22	0.28	-0.62	0.24
Class	Volition	Values	-0.25	-0.25	0.09	-0.46	-0.06
Class	Volition	DW	0.34	0.50	0.12	0.31	0.77

To prepare the variables for the regression models, I computed a composite score for social class using the three indicator variables comprising latent construct – income, childhood social class, and current social class. To ensure equivalency of scales, which could affect the analyses, I standardized the composite social class score, the work volition scale score, and all potential moderator variables. Descriptive statistics for the potential moderator variables prior to standardization are presented in Table 7. In the

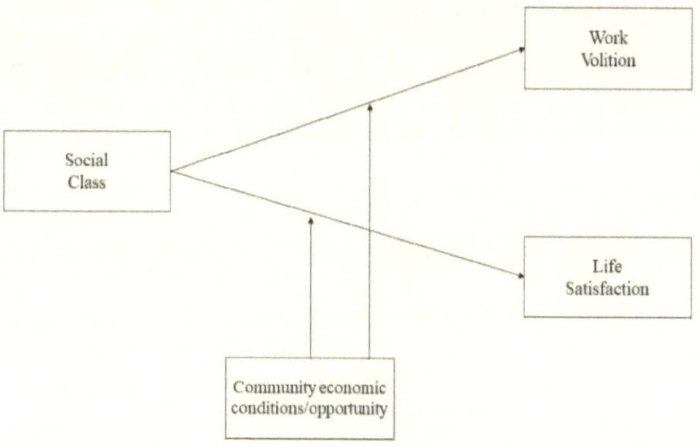

Figure 6. Portion of full structural model from Figure 1 highlighting two moderation pathways.

first model, I regressed the composite social class variable, particular moderator variable, and an interaction term (e.g. social class x poverty rates) on work volition. Figure 7 depicts this general approach. I ran this model several times, only substituting different moderator variables listed in Table 7. No moderation analyses yielded significant effects for the interaction term in these models, which would have indicated potential moderation. In a second model, I regressed the composite social class variable, particular moderation variable, and an interaction term on life satisfaction, and repeated the same process described for model 1. Again, no interaction terms appeared significant.

In light of these null results, despite a breadth of literature documenting the impact of community context on individuals, I ran further analyses using a categorical version of the moderator. To do this, I divided the community opportunity and economic conditions index scores into three categories: those in approximately the top 25%, those in the bottom 25% and those in the middle. I then created two dummy variables – one comparing the top 25% to the middle group, and one comparing the bottom 25% to the middle group. I ran the two models again, including social class, the two dummy variables, and two interaction terms (e.g. social x each dummy variable). This approach attempted to account for the possibility that the relationship between social class and work volition might differ based on levels of community economic conditions and opportunity. Despite this approach, the models still did not yield any significant moderation effects.

Table 7

Descriptive Statistics of Moderator Variables (n=816)

Variable	Mean	SD	Min	Max	Skewness	Kurtosis
Economic	183.65	110.85	1	386	0.06	0.15
Unemploy	4.12	1.16	2	19.2	3.69	36.76
Income	52,886.76	15,333.36	24,523.17	11,4811.3	1.66	3.36
Poverty	15.43	5.31	4	53.3	0.59	3.38
80/20	4.79	0.82	3.29	8.83	1.69	0.31

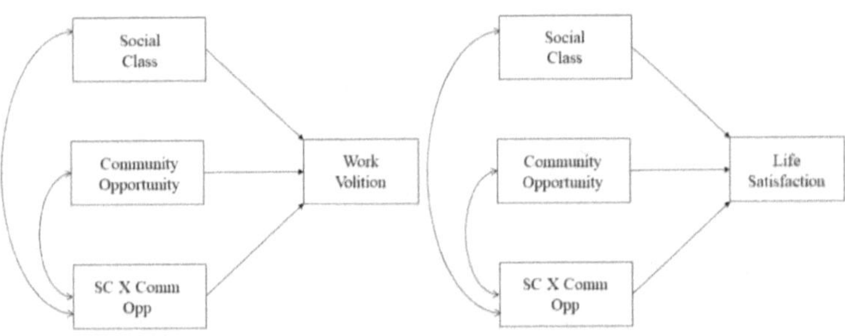

Figure 7. Regression models highlighting the two moderation analyses with manifest variables.

Results of Hypothesis Tests

In general, hypotheses related to the direct and indirect pathways in the full SEM model were mixed. Results of the hypothesis testing vary depending on which SEM model is considered. The main difference in SEM models is the inclusion of a global decent work factor in the second. For parsimony, answers to the hypotheses are based on use of the five-factor construct. However, Tables 8 (direct effects) and 9 (indirect effects) compare hypothesized pathways in each model.

1. Social class will be positively associated with the outcomes of life satisfaction, decent work and work volition.

    a. As hypothesized, social class was positively associated with life satisfaction.

    b. Within the full structural model, I estimated pathways from social class to each of the five components of decent work. After controlling for work volition, social class positively predicted the Healthcare component and negatively predicted the Rest component of decent work.

    c. As hypothesized, social class was positively associated with work volition.

2. Work volition will mediate the relationship from social class to decent work.

    a. Based on significance testing of the indirect regression coefficients, the pathways from social class to all five components of decent work via work volition were significant. By comparing indirect effects to direct and total effects, work volition appeared to partially mediate the pathways to the

Healthcare, and to fully mediate the pathways to Safety, Compensation, Rest, and Values.

3. Decent work will be positively associated with life satisfaction.

    a. The Compensation and Values components positively predicted life satisfaction.

Table 8

Hypothesis testing from structural model		
Hypothesized Direct Pathways	Supported?	
	Five-factor Structure	**Bifactor Structure**
1. Class → Work Volition	Supported	Supported
2. Class → Safe	X	X
3. Class → Health	Supported	Supported
4. Class → Compensation	X	X
5. Class → Rest	X	Supported
6. Class → Values	X	X
7. Class → Global DW	Not tested	X
8. Class → Life Satisfaction	Supported	X
8. Work volition → Safe	Supported	X
9. Work volition → Health	Supported	X
10. Work volition → Compensation	Supported	X
11. Work volition → Rest	Supported	X
12. Work volition → Values	Supported	X
13. Work volition → global DW	Not tested	Supported
14. Safe → Life Satisfaction	X	X
15. Health → Life Satisfaction	Supported	X
16. Compensation → Life Satisfaction	Supported	X
17. Rest → Life Satisfaction	X	X
18. Values → Life Satisfaction	Supported	X
19. DW → Life Satisfaction	Not tested	Supported

4. Community economic conditions and opportunity will moderate the relationship between social class and work volition.

    a. This hypothesis was unsupported.

5. Community economic conditions and opportunity will moderate the pathway from social class to life satisfaction.

a. This hypothesis was unsupported.

Table 9

Hypothesis testing from structural model

Hypothesized Indirect Pathways		Supported?	
		Five-Factor Model	Bifactor Model
1.	Class → Work Volition → Safe	Supported	X
2.	Class → Work Volition → Health	Supported	X
3.	Class → Work Volition → Compensation	Supported	X
4.	Class → Work Volition → Rest	Supported	X
5.	Class → Work Volition → Values	Supported	X
6.	Class → Work Volition → Global DW	NA	X

Chapter 5

Discussion

The positive impact of work on well-being is clear (Paul & Moser, 2009), and unfortunately the career development field has historically neglected to study these fundamental aspects of life within society's most vulnerable populations (Blustein, 2006; 2013). Amidst the COVID-19 pandemic, unemployment rates in the U.S. are increasing rapidly, with most recent data estimating nearly one in four Americans filing for unemployment (Cheung, 2020). While the pandemic has undoubtedly impacted the work lives of the majority of Americans in some capacity, it is illuminating vulnerabilities to precarious and indecent working conditions already facing low-income and minority populations in the working world. This environment necessitates comprehensive exploration of individuals' psychological experience of work and well-being, particularly for those already experiencing instability and uncertainty. Although data for the present study was collected prior to the pandemic, the study sought to investigate pathways by which individual economic constraints impact work and work-related variables, in addition to well-being, and the role of community economic conditions and opportunity in these relationships.

Utilizing the PWT model through an SEM framework, the present study builds upon a body of research examining the construct of decent work and its proposed predictors and outcomes. Furthermore, the study attempted to explore the role of the hypothesized moderator of economic conditions. By testing both five-factor and bifactor decent work latent structures in the full model, the analyses have contributed to understanding the multidimensional nature of decent work by providing evidence for both independent functioning of the subcomponents of decent work and a global decent work construct. This chapter will first summarize major study results before contextualizing them with extant research on PWT. Subsequent sections will then discuss implications for research, practice and policy, before concluding with a discussion of study limitations.

Summary of Findings

The present study utilized latent structural equation modeling to test several hypothesized tenets of the PWT model involving the latent constructs of social class, work volition, decent work and well-being (measured as life satisfaction). Modeling analyses using both correlational and bifactor decent work structures produced good fitting SEM models. In both models, social class directly predicted work volition, as well as the Healthcare and Rest components of DW, although the relationship to the latter was negative. In the five-factor model, social class also predicted life satisfaction and work volition predicted all five components of DW. These relationships did not remain significant when using the bifactor structure, but work volition did predict the global DW variable. In the five-factor model, the Compensation and Values components significantly predicted life satisfaction. Again, these effects disappeared when using the bifactor model and instead, the global factor predicted life satisfaction. Controlling for global DW, the insignificance of work volition's effect on the discrete components of DW and of these components' effects on life satisfaction suggests that variance in the discrete components in the first model was absorbed by the variance related to the global

DW factor in the second model. Similarly, global DW appeared to diminish social class' effect on life satisfaction, as evidenced by its drop in significance.

Mediational analyses were conducted with both models to explore the indirect effects of work volition. In the first model, work volition appeared to partially mediate the relationship between social class and Healthcare and to fully mediate the relationship between social class and the other four components of DW. In the second model, work volition appeared to fully mediate the relationship between social class and decent work. Indirect effects also appeared significant, but negative, in mediational paths to Healthcare and Values components.

Following overall SEM model testing and mediational analyses, two sets of moderation analyses were conducted to determine if economic conditions and community opportunity moderated the relationship between social class and work volition, and between social class and life satisfaction. Neither set of analyses yielded significant moderation effects. In the sections that follow, the results from the present study are considered in relation to theoretical premises and findings that are consistent and divergent with those reported here.

Convergent Findings

A number of studies have tested the PWT model to better understand the role of decent work in people's lives in several communities, including but not limited to, LGBTQ (Douglass et al., 2017), racial and ethnic minority (Duffy et al., 2018; Duffy et al., 2019), women (England et al., 2020), low-income Turkish (Kozan et al., 2019), Chinese (Wang et al., 2019) and Korean (Kim et al., 2019) populations. Broadly speaking and consistent with this research, the present study found the portions of the PWT model tested within an SEM framework to be a good fit for the data. Studies to date have utilized varying DW structures in measurement models (i.e. higher-order, five-factor, bifactor) but, with the exception of one pathway in Duffy, Gensmer et al. (2019), have ultimately examined hypothesized pathways using a global decent work factor. Conversely, the present study examined hypothesized relationships using a global decent work variable in conjunction with the five subfactors (bifactor model) and with these subfactors in isolation (five-factor model). The latter approach adds to growing knowledge of how distinct aspects of DW function within the PWT model. Moreover, the bifactor model approach reveals how these components function amid shared variance from the global factor.

Studies utilizing a global DW factor have yielded mixed results for a direct relationship between economic constraints and decent work, with some finding support for a direct relationship (Douglass et al., 2017; Kim et al., 2019; Kozan et al., 2019); the results from the current study are consistent with other studies that did not observe this direct relationship (e.g., Duffy et al., 2018; Duffy et al., 2019). Consistent with some of the most well-supported tenets of PWT, the present model revealed an indirect relationship between social class and decent work via work volition, as well as a direct relationship between work volition and decent work (Douglass et al., 2017; Duffy et al., 2018; Duffy et al., 2019; England et al., 2020 Kim et al., 2019; Kozan et al., 2019). These findings demonstrate the role of social class in shaping one's perceptions of choice in career decision-making, and the powerful impact a sense of volition in turn has on securing decent work. Similar to the Kozan et al. (2019) study which examined the direct impact of decent work on life satisfaction, the current study corroborates this positive predictive pathway. Notably, the PWT model does not include a direct pathway from social class to life satisfaction in its tenets, but implies an indirect pathway from the predictor to one of the final outcomes via several mediating constructs, including decent work. However, given the breadth of research on social class as a social determinant of health (Solar & Irwin, 2018), the direct pathway was incorporated and supported in the present study.

While researchers have mostly examined hypothesized pathways with global decent work, Duffy, Gensmer et al. (2019) also specified and detected a significant direct effect for social class on Healthcare. The present study supports this direct predictive relationship from social class to Healthcare. Although not within an SEM framework, evidence from latent profile analyses (LPA) also highlight initial support for the discrete functioning of DW components (Blustein et al., under review; Kim et al., 2020). In their study, Kim et al. (2020) found that levels of the Healthcare component differentiated two of five major profiles. Coupled with these prior studies (Duffy, Gensmer et al., 2019; Kim et al., 2020), the present study suggests that access to healthcare is a defining feature of individuals' experiences and perceptions of decent work in the U.S.

Taken together, the present study substantiates the proposed linear pathway along which social class predicts work volition, which in turn predicts global DW, and ultimately determines life satisfaction. Additionally, current findings support a direct relationship from social class to Healthcare.

Divergent Findings

This section outlines unexpected results and attempts to explicate them through methodological and theoretical considerations to enrich theoretical premises and deepen understanding. Importantly, the PWT-hypothesized tenets do not explicitly relate to specific pathways with the components of DW. Therefore, divergent findings are considered through application of PWT according to its conceptualization of global DW functioning. Additionally, little research has yet examined the individual components within the PWT model, making direct comparisons to other empirical evidence limited. The following section first addresses deviant findings related to the social class variable and the DW components, followed by predictors of life satisfaction, and concludes with moderation. The section concludes with a summary.

Pathway from social class to DW components

Few known studies have examined the direct effects of social class on the five components of decent work through SEM, although some researchers have examined these components through profile analyses (Blustein et al., under review; Kim et al., 2020). Contrary to theoretical tenets that social class would directly predict all five components of DW, social class positively predicted the Healthcare and negatively predicted the Rest components of DW. Put another way, individuals with higher social class backgrounds were more likely to report having decent work with adequate healthcare benefits, but less likely to report having work that allows them time to for non-work activities and rest. While inconsistent with the direction of original hypothesized propositions, the negative association between social class and Rest underscores the multidimensionality of DW and the possibility that this relationship may not be linear. For instance, an individual belonging to a higher social class may be in a higher level position with a number of adequate conditions, but given their level of responsibility or pressure to perform, may not be able to and/or feel like they can take time off. On the other end of the spectrum, someone with very limited economic resources may be more likely to have a job that lacks benefits such as paid leave and cannot afford to take time off.

Several possible methodological and theoretical considerations might help to explain why social class did not predict the other components of DW. The present study specified the latent construct of economic constraints using the indicators of median annual income, current social class, and childhood social class. Within this latent structure, the factor loading for childhood social class was somewhat low, albeit still acceptable. Additionally, PWT researchers have not typically used childhood social class as an indicator for the economic constraints predictor variable. Furthermore, a majority of studies thus far have used a variety of indicators for defining proxy variables to represent the economic constraints construct, most often using some combination of the MacArthur Social Standing ladder (Adler et al., 2000), current social class, and annual household income. These variations in measurement pose a challenge to assessing the predictive nature of economic constraints in the PWT model. In an attempt to remedy this issue, researchers have developed a scale of lifetime economic constraints (Duffy, Gensmer et al., 2019). While the scale demonstrated good internal and construct validity in the scale development study, it did not directly predict access to decent work, leaving researchers to question this proposed tenet of the PWT model (Duffy, Gesner et al., 2019). Further possible theoretical considerations for conceptualizing the economic constraints construct are discussed below.

In addition to potential measurement issues of the social class construct, measurement limitations of the decent work components might help explain why the present study failed to demonstrate hypothesized directions to and from distinct decent work components. Although the present study found that global decent work predicted life satisfaction, no known studies have examined how the components of DW impact this outcome. Whereas PWT hypothesizes that each component would positively predict life satisfaction, the present study found positive predictive relationships for only Compensation and Values, meaning that participants that report having adequate compensation and congruent values with their work, also report greater levels of life satisfaction. Of note, an item on the Rest and an item on the Compensation components significantly cross-loaded with one and two other components, respectively. Additionally, the item in the Rest component was only mildly correlated with the other two items in this component. Findings related to correlations among items are difficult, given that recent publications have not reported on this level of detail.

Predictors of life satisfaction

In addition to failing to predict all components of decent work, social class did not significantly predict life satisfaction, after including global DW in the model. Again, this null result may be in part because the variance of global DW masked the variance from social class. The aforementioned measurement limitations related to social class may also have contributed to weakening the potential variance from social class. Alternately, given the linear pathway from the start to the end of the model through work volition and decent work, global decent work may function as a mediator. Namely, people with higher social class backgrounds are more likely to have decent work, and decent work then leads to being more satisfied with life. Again, while PWT does not postulate about this potential mediation pathway, it is implied in how the model is structured. Therefore, future studies utilizing a similar set of variables might test for mediation effects of DW.

As mentioned above, the PWT model hypothesizes that decent work influences life satisfaction through PWT needs satisfaction. Researchers have begun to explore these mediational pathways (Autin et al., 2019; Duffy, Kim et al., 2019), but again considered the pathway from a global decent work factor to life satisfaction via needs satisfaction. Notably, Duffy, Kim et al. (2019) found that the PWT needs fully mediated the pathway from decent work to well-being. Thus, future research should explore this mediational pathway from the individual components of DW to life satisfaction through PWT needs satisfaction.

Moderating effects

Researchers have devoted less attention to testing the potential moderating role of economic conditions in the PWT model. While PWT scholars refer to unemployment rates and economic recessions as examples of macro-level economic conditions (Duffy et al., 2016), mechanisms for examining these factors are in their infancy, although PWT calls for interdisciplinary approaches. Whereas all other constructs in the PWT model are analyzed at the individual level, and have been assessed through self-report thus far, the economic conditions moderator serves as a macro-level factor in the model and accordingly, warrants the need for innovative analytic methods. The present study focused on economic conditions and community opportunity at the county-level. Contrary to PWT tenets and a breadth of research demonstrating the impact of community economic conditions on individual well-being (Abramovitz & Albercht,

2013; Ali et al., 2017; Wilson, 2017)), the present study did not reveal significant findings. Several methodological issues and theoretical perspectives may serve to elucidate this null finding.

While psychologists are increasingly attending to the importance of community context in individuals' psychological and vocational well-being ((Blustein, Ali et al., 2019; Bronfenbrenner & Morris, 2006), one potential explanation is that one's social location (social class in this case) and personal economic resources play a much greater role in their sense of volition and life satisfaction than that of their communities (Bronfenbrenner & Morris, 2006). Alternatively, specifying community factors as a moderator in the model may not accurately portray the relationship among individual economic resources, community economic conditions, and psychological outcomes. Rather, community opportunity might shape, or predict, an individual's access to resources and subsequent social class to a greater degree than it does as a moderator in the relationship between current social class and work volition/life satisfaction.

Although the data appear to represent varying levels of economic conditions, aspects of geographic diversity may affect people more than economic conditions. For instance, a county in Atlanta, GA and a county in rural South Dakota may score similarly on indicators of economic conditions. However, the participants in these counties, controlling for personal economic resources, may experience these economic conditions quite differently. For instance, the person in Atlanta may be able to work in, or send their child to school, in a neighboring county, whereas the individual in the rural county may not have access. Additionally, two participants in neighboring, albeit very differently resourced communities, may have more similar experiences than two participants in similarly resourced communities on opposite sides of the country. Although there are numerous ways in which communities differ culturally, historically, and economically, among other things, one means to better capture community effects would be to compare rural and urban communities. Thus, integrating strictly economic conditions at the county-level, cross-sectionally, may not be the best methodological approach for examining how economic conditions impact the relationship between social class and work volition, and further approaches should be explored. For instance, researchers who have detected community level effects in social mobility and well-being have utilized longitudinal, quasi-experimental designs (Chetty et al., 2018). As such, the way in which community effects was defined and measured in the present study may be too broad and may attenuate the impacts of challenging social and economic conditions.

Within the spirit of MacLachlan's (2014) charge for psychologists to move beyond individual-levels of investigation, the present study attempted to integrate macro-level factors (i.e. county-level data) and psychological factors in its design. This attempt was further prompted by PWT scholars' (Duffy et al., 2016) insistence on interdisciplinary approaches to more fully examine the PWT model, and their conceptualization of a potential moderator as a macro-level variable. Despite inconclusive findings for the role of economic conditions as a moderating variable in the current study, future research should continue to employ innovative methods and to foster interdisciplinary collaboration in order to better understand the role of systemic factors in work and well-being, according to the essence of PWT.

Summary

The present study contributes further empirical support for previous findings related to the functioning of a global construct. Namely, social class appears to indirectly predict DW through work volition and DW positively relates to life satisfaction. When examining discrete DW components in tandem with a global construct, social class positively predicts Healthcare and negatively predicts Rest, attesting to the uniqueness of variance in these components. Furthermore, decent work appears to mediate the relationship between social class and life satisfaction, further demonstrating the compelling role of decent work in people's lives. Comparing results from models utilizing the bifactor and five-factor DW structures suggests that utility of these structure will depend upon the particular research question.

Research and theoretical implications

Results of the present study contribute to the growing body of research that utilizes the PWT model to better understand the importance of decent work in people's lives, particularly for those from marginalized backgrounds. Furthermore, these findings underscore the multidimensionality of decent work and the reality that individuals may experience decent work in some areas, but not in others. Adding to prior research, the present study also supports a holistic decent work construct. Taken together, either DW structure might be employed in future research on decent work, depending on the particular aim of the study.

Due to the present study's mixed findings related to the five components of decent work, future research should investigate how proposed predictors and outcomes function in relation to each component. One means toward this aim is to use the correlational structure of DW, which may require larger sample sizes, given increased parameters (England et al., 2019). Several studies assessing the cross-cultural validity of the DWS have found slightly better fitting measurement models with the correlational structure in comparison to the bifactor structure, further conveying its potential utility (Buyukgoze-Kavas & Autin, 2019; Ferreira et al., 2019).

As more researchers utilize the correlational structure to examine the heterogeneity of DW, continuing to attend to the latent construction of the DW subcomponents will be imperative, especially considering that each subcomponent is currently defined by the minimum recommended three items as indicators. As previously mentioned, two items on the DWS appeared to cross-load with other components, which may threaten the discreteness of these components. When using the DWS in a cross-cultural context, Nam and Kim's (2019) study produced a Cronbach's alpha for the Rest subscale of 0.58. Furthermore, when examining factor loadings of items on the global construct, some components appear to load more strongly on the global factor than others, suggesting that the higher loading subcomponents may be contributing most to the variance in the global factor. Taken together, researchers might consider exploring additional items to bolster the robustness of these constructs in future research.

As previously mentioned, researchers have used a variety of indicators to represent the economic constraints construct. To enhance consistency in research, Duffy, Gensmer et al. (2019) have developed the Economic Constraints Scale (ECS) for use in the PWT model. However, results for the hypothesized pathway from economic constraints to DW remain inconclusive. The construct is defined as "limited economic resources (e.g., household income, family wealth) which represent a critical barrier to securing decent work" (Duffy et al., 2016, p. 133). The ECS intends to encompass the cumulative effects of limited economic resources across the lifespan on access to decent work, as opposed to just at present (Duffy, Gensmer et al., 2019). While the proposed mechanism of work volition by which economic constraints impact access to decent work has amassed substantial empirical support, researchers might continue to expand their conceptualization of other means through which economic constraints influence access to decent work. For instance, limited financial resources may inhibit social capital and educational opportunities, leading to less decent work. Therefore, future research might explore additional mechanisms through which economic resources and social class impact decent work. As research on the distinct components of DW grows, studies might also investigate whether indicators of social class and economic constraints impact these components differentially.

The present study highlights the potential to utilize a bifactor or five-factor model to answer particular research questions. In moving forward with a five-factor model, researchers might seek to expand upon measures of the individual components, as well as the economic constraints construct. Furthermore, researchers might consider the utility of estimating both global and individual factors in hypothesized pathways, as well as how to conceptualize the shared variance of the global construct, after partitioning variance of the distinct components.

Practice and Policy Implications

The current study reinforces the critical role of work in well-being (Paul & Moser, 2009), in addition to social class's influence in securing decent work both directly and in shaping perceptions of career choice. Therefore, attending to the securement of economic resources and the decency of work is critical for counseling psychologists on both individual and systemic levels. As such, the following section will outline implications for counseling before positing possible systemic interventions that psychologists can take in accordance to a vocational psychology social justice agenda (Blustein, Ali, & Flores, 2019).

Counseling

Present empirical evidence that social class negatively impacts general decent work and life satisfaction highlights the need for therapists to integrate mental health and career counseling in their work. These findings further underscore the interwoven nature of well-being and work, and as such, counselors should avoid making artificial distinctions and incorporate elements of both in their practice to best serve their clients (Blustein, 2006; 2008). To this end, the PWF is relevant, as it was developed to advance an inclusive counseling agenda infusing traditional career development approaches and mental health counseling, as needed, to meet the needs of all those who work and want to work (Blustein, 2006; 2013).

Following the guidelines of PWF and more recent applications (Blustein, Kenny, Autin, & Duffy, 2019), counselors should assess clients' need fulfillment in the working context, including survival, relational, social contribution, and self-determination. To enact meaningful change, it is critical to attend to both survival and self-determination in order to address immediate needs and support a long-term goal to ultimately achieve meaningful work. Within this same vein, the present study demonstrates the importance of assessing various components of decent work with clients to better understand what aspects are most essential for them to feel fulfilled and supported. For example, someone might have access to healthcare benefits through a partner and therefore this element is less critical, whereas having adequate time off is crucial given this same individuals' young children. Of note, the Healthcare component emerged as linked to social class, signifying the decreased likelihood of individuals with lower economic resources securing work that provides adequate healthcare. Within the context of the aforementioned cross-cultural studies on the DWS, this finding appears specific to the U.S. context as most of the countries in these studies have a government-run healthcare system and therefore fewer participants outside of the U.S. cited healthcare as an element of decent work. However, for counselors in the US, exploring clients' access to healthcare appears essential (Kim et al., 2020). Therefore, counselors should work with clients to find ways to access adequate healthcare through work, or to obtain it through other avenues (such as government-sponsored programs).

In addition to the importance of healthcare in people's lives, rest and time off also emerged as significantly intertwined with social class. Interestingly, higher levels of social class appeared negatively related to having adequate time to rest and time off. In general, this finding signifies the importance of exploring a client's ability to take time off from work. Depending on the type of occupation or the workplace culture of an organization, an individual may be deterred from taking time off. Alternatively, their organization may not provide adequate provisions for rest and time off. Regardless of the cause, it appears critical that counselors discuss a client's benefits in this domain, their feelings related to utilizing existing benefits, and in general, their needs related to this component of decent work.

Following an examination of a clients' needs, counselors can explore how they envision varying components of decent work meeting these needs. These discussions can then enable clients to build a corresponding, individualized decent work agenda, which serves as one means for fostering agentic action (Blustein, Kenny, Autin et al., 2019; Richardson, 2000). Additionally, engaging in critical consciousness raising discussions can lead clients to reflect critically on how limiting opportunity structures and structural oppression may be impacting their experience of, and access to, decent work (Diemer et al., 2016; Freire, 2007). These reflective dialogues may help clients better understand their perceptions of choice in career-decision making and when coupled with taking critical actions, bolster their work volition, which appears instrumental in attaining decent work. Furthermore, increasing critical consciousness can help alleviate self-blame that clients might experience based on negative work experiences, as they are better able to externalize the cause of these negative experiences (Sharone, 2014).

Policy

Given that systemic forces shape individuals' access to economic resources and decent work, fostering agentic action on an individual level is not sufficient to truly transform inequity in the world of work; consistent with PWT and broader social justice movements, counseling psychologists must seek to instigate structural change (Duffy et al., 2016). Where possible, psychologists can pursue avenues to advocate for government policies that regulate employers' implementation of human capital practices to ensure employees' work is decent. Organizations such as the ILO and United Nations have declared decent work a human right and PWT scholars align with this agenda (Blustein, 2019; Blustein, Kenny, Di Fabio, & Guichard, 2019); as such, psychologists can collaborate with these types of organizations to develop alliances and conjoint initiatives that will enhance the work lives of people across the globe. With increasing short-term contract and precarious work, workers often do not receive work security or benefits, and therefore, government policies are critical for safeguarding these workers' rights. Given the current study's finding that healthcare is a salient element of decent work, systemic healthcare reform in the U.S. could meet this essential need. For instance, providing government-funded healthcare to all would eliminate equities in access to healthcare, which have been largely dependent on employers to provide.

Grounded in results related to rest and time off, government and organizational policies should focus on ensuring workers receive adequate paid leave. Again, individuals engaged in contract or gig work are unlikely to receive these benefits and depending on their economic resources, may not be able to afford to take unpaid time off.

Limitations

Although the current study substantiates and builds upon prior empirical support for the PWT model, it is not without its limitations. Whereas PWT scholars conceptualized the predictor of economic constraints as the experience of having limited economic resources across the lifespan, the present study utilized the proxy variable of social class to represent this construct, and thus, may not have fully captured the construct. Additionally, while participants' perceptions of social class might encapsulate some form of class-based marginalization, the present study did not include the second major contextual predictor of marginalization in the model. Given PWT's aim to represent marginalized communities' experiences, the exclusion of a marginalization measure does not allow for an examination of how marginalization based on race, ethnicity, sexual orientation, gender identity, and many other social identities, impacts individuals' access to decent work, which is likely instrumental

The economic conditions moderator variable also has a few notable weaknesses. Two county-level measures comprised the moderation variables – an economic composite index and an overall opportunity index. The measures were created by Opportunity Nation (2017), which collated data from a variety of publically available sources, such as the Census Bureau and the BLS. The data for indicators constituting these indices were collected at varying times between 2011 and 2017, depending on both the data source and the county. Thus, the individual level data in the study, which was collected from Spring 2018 – Spring 2019, does not match participants' associated county-level data. This incongruence in time limits inferences using these variables. Moreover, the individual- and county-level data were matched using participant IP addresses, which assumes that participants' IP addresses indicate where they live. However, it is plausible that participants may have completed the survey from a device at a workplace, an educational setting, or a library, among other possible locations. Importantly, these locations may be in a different county than that of the participant's home, and thus, this potential discrepancy reveals another source of error.

Along with needing up-to-date data to more accurately capture community context, unemployment rates came from the Bureau of Labor Statistics (2017). Of note, researchers have cited that BLS unemployment rates are likely an underestimate of those in need of work (Duffy et al., 2016). For instance, there have been lower levels or labor market participation since 2007, which suggests that there are likely three to four percent fewer people working that is not captured in unemployment rates (Duffy et al., 2016). In a similar vein, unemployment rates may not adequately reflect reality as economic crises related to the COVID-19 pandemic continue. Hence, as vocational psychology researchers seek to investigate work in the midst of, and following, the pandemic, they will need to view these rates with caution and explore other means for assessing job loss. Qualitative studies might be better suited to explore how economic recessions impact workers' psychological experiences, given the lack of extant research in this area.

Although researchers have found MTurk samples to be as representative as undergraduate student or community samples, the sample is not without its limitations (Goodman et al., 2013). Research suggests that participants recruited through MTurk tend to have higher levels of education than the general public, which was true of this study's sample. Additionally, the Mean age of the present sample was 35.7, thus representing a slightly younger sample than would be expected of the working-age population (BLS, 2019). Furthermore, the sample includes a greater ratio of male to female participants, 62 and 38 percent respectively, compared to the gender breakdown of the general population (U.S. Census Bureau, 2019). The use of online sampling excludes individuals without access to the internet, and likely those more vulnerable to lacking decent work. Lastly, the data collected focused on people experiencing some level of precarity in their work lives, which represents a sub-section of the population. These potential limitations to a representative sample inhibit the generalizability of this study.

Finally, because the present study utilized a cross-sectional, correlational design, casual inferences cannot be made. To confirm hypothesized directional relationships among the variables, longitudinal studies are necessary. Additionally, with the exception of the economic conditions variable, all measures were collected through self-report and further research should expand upon sources of individual data.

Despite these limitations, the present study's inclusion of two SEM models mitigate some of these limitations. By utilizing varying structures of decent work, I was able to observe which relationships remained significant regardless of structure, providing a mechanism for corroborating results within the sample. Additionally, by examining all three scale structures through CFA, multiple full measurement and SEM models, I was able to closely observe some of the psychometric properties of the various DW measures and highlight potential areas to make these measures more robust.

Conclusions

The present study sought to better understand how social class and decent work function in tandem, along with perceptions of choice in work and overall life satisfaction in a national adult sample of 816, geographically representative of the U.S. population. Results reinforce the critical role of work in well-being, along with the importance of economic resources in securing decent work. Furthermore, the study reveals the array of conditions necessary for ensuring that work is decent, as well as a more nuanced understanding that decent work is not a uniform entity, but rather a unique experience, requiring a comprehensive, person-centered approach. Given the integral role of work in psychological health and social mobility, decent work is a bare minimum human right in the pursuit of social justice. As such, counseling psychologists must continue to advocate for systemic interventions and expansive policy reform in order to ensure decent work for all. As researchers seek to instigate systemic change, the PWT model appears fitting for understanding how work and mental health are intertwined, and for guiding research agendas. These explorations will be crucial, particularly in light of the widespread impact of the COVID-19 crisis and its' exceedingly detrimental impact on individuals already facing immense injustice.

References

Abramovitz, M., & Albrecht, J. (2013). The community loss index: A new social indicator. *Social Service Review, 87*(4), 677-724.

Adler, N. E., Epel, E. S., Castellazzo, G., & Ickovics, J. R. (2000). Relationship of subjective and objective social status with psychological and physiological functioning: Preliminary data in healthy white women. *Health Psychology, 19*, 586 –592.

Aldrich, D. P., & Meyer, M. A. (2015). Social capital and community resilience. *American Behavioral Scientist, 59*(2), 254-269.

Ali, S. R. (2013). Poverty, social class, and working. In D. L. Blustein (Ed.), *The Oxford handbook of the psychology of working* (pp. 127–140). New York, NY: Oxford University Press.

Ali, S. R., Brown, S. D., & Loh, Y. (2017). Project HOPE: Evaluation of health science career education programming for rural Latino and European American youth. *Career Development Quarterly, 65*, 57-71.

Ananat, E. O., Gassman-Pines, A., Francis, D. V., & Gibson-Davis, C. M. (2017). Linking job loss, inequality, mental health, and education. *Science, 356*(6343), 1127-1128.

Autin, K. L., Duffy, R. D., Blustein, D. L., Gensmer, N. P., Douglass, R. P., England, J. W., & Allan, B. A. (2019). The development and initial validation of need satisfaction scales within the psychology of working theory. *Journal of Counseling Psychology, 66*(2), 195-209.

Baron, R. M., & Kenny, D. A. (1986). The moderator-mediator variable distinction in social psychological research: Conceptual, strategic, and statistical considerations. *Journal of Personality and Social Psychology, 51*, 1173-1182.

Benzell, S. G., Kotlikoff, L. J., LaGarda, G., & Sachs, J. D. (2015). Robots are us: Some economics of human replacement. Working paper, National Bureau for Economic Research. Retrieved from http://www.bu.edu/econ/files/2015/05/Robots_Are_Us_3-29-20151.pdf

Blustein, D. L. & Duffy, R. D. (in press). Psychology of Working Theory. In S.D. Brown and R.W. Lent (Eds.), *Career development and counseling: Putting theory and research to work* (3rd ed). Hoboken, NJ: Wiley.

Blustein, D. L. (2006). *The psychology of working: A new perspective for career development, counseling, and public policy.* New York, NY: Routledge.

Blustein, D. L. (2008). The role of work in psychological health and well-being: A conceptual, historical, and public policy perspective. *American Psychologist, 63*(4), 228.

Blustein, D. L. (Ed.) (2013). *The Oxford handbook of the psychology of working.* New York, NY: Oxford University Press.

Blustein, D. L. (2019). Developing, validating, and testing improved measures within the psychology of working theory. *Journal of Vocational Behavior, 112*, 199-215.

Blustein, D. L., Ali, S. R., & Flores, L. Y. (2019). Vocational psychology: Expanding the vision and enhancing the impact. *The Counseling Psychologist, 47*(2), 166-221.

Blustein, D. L., Kenna, A. C., Gill, N., & Devoy, J. E. (2008). The psychology of

working: A new framework for counseling practice and public policy. *The Career

Development Quarterly, 56,* 294–308.

Blustein, D.L., Kenny, M.E., Autin, K.L., & Duffy, R.D. (2019). Psychology of working

in practice: A theory of change for new era. *Career Development Quarterly, 67,*

236-254.

Blustein, D. L., Kenny, M. E., Di Fabio, A., & Guichard, J. (2019). Expanding the impact

of the psychology of working: Engaging psychology in the struggle for decent

work and human rights. *Journal of Career Assessment, 27,* 3-28.

Blustein, D. L., McWhirter, E. H., & Perry, J. C. (2005). An emancipatory

communitarian approach to vocational development theory, research, and

practice. *The Counseling Psychologist, 33,* 141–179.

Blustein, D. L., Olle, C., Connors-Kellgren, A., & Diamonti, A. J. (2016). Decent Work:

A psychological perspective. *Frontiers in Psychology, 7,* 407.

Bronfenbrenner, U., & Morris, P. A. (2006). The bioecological model of human

development. In W. Damon & R. M. Lerner (Eds.), *Handbook of child

psychology: Vol. 1. Theoretical models of human development* (6th ed., pp. 793–

828). Hoboken, NJ: Wiley.

Brown, M. T. (2004). The career development influence of family of origin:

Considerations of race/ethnic group membership and class. *The Counseling

Psychologist, 32*(4), 587-595.

Brown, M. T., Fukunaga, C., Umemoto, D., & Wicker, L. (1996). Annual Review, 1990-
1996: Social class, work, and retirement behavior. *Journal of Vocational
Behavior, 49*, 159-189.

Bor, J. (2017). Diverging life expectancy and voting patterns in the 2016 U.S.
Presidential election. *American Journal of Public Health, 107*(10), 1560-1562.

Buhrmester, M., Kwang, T. & Gosling, S. D. (2011). Amazon's Mechanical Turk: A new
source of inexpensive, yet high-quality, data? *Perspectives on Psychological
Science, 6*, 3–5.

Bureau of Labor Statistics (2018). Local Area Unemployment Statistics and news
releases. Retrieved from http://www.bls.gov/lau/

Chetty, R., Grusky, D., Hell, M., Hendren, N., Manduca, R., & Narang, J. (2017). The
fading American dream: Trends in absolute income mobility since
1940. *Science, 356*(6336), 398-406.

Chetty, R., & Hendren, N. (2016). *The impacts of neighborhoods on intergenerational
mobility II: County-level estimates* (No. w23002). National Bureau of Economic
Research.

Chetty, R., & Hendren, N. (2018). The impacts of neighborhoods on intergenerational
mobility I: Childhood exposure effects. *The Quarterly Journal of
Economics, 133*(3), 1107-1162.

Chetty, R., Hendren, N., & Katz, L. F. (2016). The effects of exposure to better
neighborhoods on children: New evidence from the Moving to Opportunity
experiment. *American Economic Review, 106*(4), 855-902.

Cheung, F., & Lucas, R. E. (2016). Income inequality is associated with stronger social comparison effects: The effect of relative income on life satisfaction. *Journal of personality and social psychology, 110*(2), 332.

Cheung, H. (2020). One in four US workers claiming jobless benefits. *British Broadcasting Corporation*. Retrieved from www.bbc.com.

Cho, S., Crenshaw, K. W., & McCall, L. (2013). Toward a field of intersectionality studies: Theory, applications, and praxis. *Signs: Journal of Women in Culture and Society, 38*(4), 785-810.

Cole, E.R. (2009). Intersectionality and research in psychology. *American Psychologist, 64*, 170–180.

Coleman, J. S., & Coleman, J. S. (1994). *Foundations of social theory*. Cambridge, MA: Harvard university press.

Costello, A. B., & Osborne, J. (2005). Best practices in exploratory factor analysis: Four recommendations for getting the most from your analysis. *Practical assessment, research, and evaluation, 10*(1), 7.

International Labour Organization. (2020). COVID-19 and the world of work Fourth edition. Retrieved from http://oit.org/wcmsp5/groups/public/---dgreports/---dcomm/documents/briefingnote/wcms_743146.pdf

Davies, J. B., Fortin, N. M., & Lemieux, T. (2017). Wealth inequality: Theory, measurement and decomposition. *Canadian Journal of Economics/Revue canadienne d'économique, 50*(5), 1224-1261.

Diemer, M. A., Mistry, R. S., Wadsworth, M. E., López, I., & Reimers, F. (2013). Best practices in conceptualizing and measuring social class in psychological research. *Analyses of Social Issues and Public Policy, 13*(1), 77-113.

Diemer, M. A., Perry, J. C., Laurenzi, C., & Torrey, C. L. (2012). The construction and initial validation of the Work Volition Scale. *Journal of Vocational Behavior, 80,* 400 – 411.

Diemer, M. A., & Ali, S. R. (2009). Integrating social class into vocational psychology: Theory and practice implications. *Journal of Career Assessment, 17,* 247–265.

Diener, E., Emmons, R. A., Larsen, R. J., & Griffin, S. (1985). The Satisfaction With Life Scale. *Journal of Personality Assessment, 49,* 71–75.

Diemer, M. A., Rapa, L. J., Voight, A. M., & McWhirter, E. H. (2016). Critical consciousness: A developmental approach to addressing marginalization and oppression. *Child Development Perspectives, 10,* 216–221.

Douglass, R. P., Velez, B. L., Conlin, S. E., Duffy, R. D., & England, J. W. (2017). Examining the psychology of working theory: Decent work among sexual minorities. *Journal of Counseling Psychology, 64*(5), 550.

Duclos, J. Y., Esteban, J., & Ray, D. (2004). Polarization: concepts, measurement, estimation. *Econometrica, 72*(6), 1737-1772.

Duffy, R.D., Allan, B.A., Blustein, D.L., England, J.W., Autin, K.L., Douglass, R.P., Ferreira, J., & Santos, E.J.R. (2017). The development and initial validation of the Decent Work Scale. *Journal of Counseling Psychology, 64*(2), 206.

Duffy, R. D., Blustein, D. L., Diemer, M. A., & Autin, K. L. (2016). The psychology of working theory. *Journal of Counseling Psychology, 63,* 127–148.

Duffy, R. D., Bott, E. M., Allan, B. A., & Torrey, C. L. (2013). Examining a model of life satisfaction among unemployed adults. *Journal of Counseling Psychology, 60*, 53– 63.

Duffy, R. D., Diemer, M. A., Perry, J. C., Laurenzi, C., & Torrey, C. L. (2012). The construction and initial validation of the Work Volition Scale. *Journal of Vocational Behavior, 80*, 400-411.

Duffy, R. D., Gensmer, N., Allan, B. A., Kim, H. J., Douglass, R. P., England, J. W., Autin, K. L., & Blustein, D. L. (2019). Developing, validating, and testing improved measures within the Psychology of Working Theory. *Journal of Vocational Behavior, 112*, 199-215.

Duffy, R. D., Douglass, R. P., & Autin, K. L. (2015). Career adaptability and academic satisfaction: Examining work volition and self-efficacy as mediators. *Journal of Vocational Behavior, 90*, 46 –54.

Duffy, R. D., Douglass, R. P., Autin, K. L., & Allan, B. A. (2015). Examining predictors of work volition among undergraduate students. *Journal of Career Assessment.*

Duffy, R. D., Kim, H. J., Gensmer, N. P., Raque-Bogdan, T. L., Douglass, R. P., England, J. W., & Buyukgoze-Kavas, A. (2019). Linking decent work with physical and mental health: A psychology of working perspective. *Journal of Vocational Behavior, 112*, 384-395.

Duffy, R. D., Velez, B. L., England, J. W., Autin, K. L., Douglass, R. P., Allan, B. A., & Blustein, D. L. (2018). An examination of the Psychology of Working Theory with racially and ethnically diverse employed adults. *Journal of counseling psychology, 65*(3), 280.

England, J. W., Duffy, R. D., Gensmer, N. P., Kim, H. J., Buyukgoze-Kavas, A., &

Larson-Konar, D. M. (2020). Women attaining decent work: The important role

of workplace climate in Psychology of Working Theory. *Journal of Counseling

Psychology, 67*(2), 251.

Fassinger, R. E. (1987). Use of structural equation modeling in counseling psychology

research. *Journal of Counseling Psychology, 34*(4), 425-436.

Festinger, L. (1954). A theory of social comparison processes. *Human Relations, 7*(2),

117-140.

Flores, L. Y., Navarro, R. L., & Ali, S. R. (2017). The state of SCCT research in relation

to social class: Future directions. *Journal of Career Assessment, 25*(1), 6-23.

Fouad, N. A., & Brown, M. T. (2000). The role of race and class in development:

Implications for counseling psychology. In S. D. Brown & R. W. Lent (Eds.),

Handbook of counseling psychology (3rd ed., pp. 379–408). New York, NY:

Wiley.

Frasquilho, D., Matos, M. G., Salonna, F., Guerreiro, D., Storti, C. C., Gaspar, T., &

Caldas-de-Almeida, J. M. (2015). Mental health outcomes in times of economic

recession: a systematic literature review. *BMC public health, 16*(1), 115.

Freire, P. (2007). *Pedagogy of the oppressed* (3rd ed.). New York, NY: The Continuum

International Publishing Group Inc.

Goodman, J.K., Cryder, C. E., & Cheema, A. (2013). Data collection in a flat world: The

strengths and weaknesses of Mechanical Turk samples. *Journal of Behavioral

Decision Making, 26*, 213–224.

Guichard, J. (2013). Career guidance, education, and dialogues for a fair and sustainable human development. In Inaugural Conference of the UNESCO Chair of Lifelong Guidance and Counselling, University of Wroclaw, Wroclaw, Poland.

Helliewell, J. F., & Huang, H. (2014). New measures of the costs of unemployment: Evidence from the subjective well-being of 3.3 million Americans. *Economic Inquiry, 52*(4), 1485-1502.

Holland, J. L. (1997). *Making vocational choices: A theory of vocational personalities and work environments* (3rd ed.). Odessa, FL: Psychological Assessment Resources.

International Labor Organization. (2008). Work of work report 2008: Income inequalities in the age of financial globalization. Retrieved from http://www.ilo.org/wcmsp5/groups/public/@dgreports/@dcomm/@publ/ documents/publication/wcms_100354.pdf

International Labor Organization. (2012). Decent work indicators: Concepts and definitions. Retrieved from http://www.ilo.org/wcmsp5/groups/ public/---dgreports/--integration/documents/publication/wcms_229374 .pdf

Jackson, D. L. (2003). Revisiting sample size and number of parameter estimates: Some support for the N: q hypothesis. *Structural equation modeling, 10*(1), 128-141.

Jorgensen, T.D., Pornprasertmanit, S., Schoemann, A.M., & Rosseel, Y. (2019). *semTools: Useful tools for structural equation modeling*. R package version 0.5-2. Retrieved from www.CRAN.R-project.org.

Kalleberg, A. L. (1989). Linking macro and micro levels: Bringing the workers back into the sociology of work. *Social Forces, 67*(3), 582.

Kalleberg, A. (2009). Precarious work, insecure workers: Employment relations in

transition. *American Sociological Review, 74,* 1-22.

Kalleberg, A. L., & Vallas, S. P. (Eds.). (2017). Probing precarious work: Theory,

research, and politics. *Research in the Sociology of Work, 31,* 1–30.

Kawachi, I., Kennedy, B. P., & Glass, R. (1999). Social capital and self-rated health: a

contextual analysis. *American journal of public health, 89*(8), 1187-1193.

Kennedy, B. P., Kawachi, I., Glass, R., & Prothrow-Stith, D. (1998). Income distribution,

socioeconomic status, and self-rated health in the United States: multilevel

analysis. *BMJ, 317*(7163), 917-921.

Kerr, W. C., Kaplan, M. S., Huguet, N., Caetano, R., Giesbrecht, N., & McFarland, B. H.

(2017). Economic recession, alcohol, and suicide rates: Comparative effects of

poverty, foreclosure, and job loss. *American Journal of Preventive

Medicine, 52*(4), 469-475.

Kim, H.J., Duffy, R.D., Lee, S., Lee, J., Lee, K.-H. (2019). Application of the psychology

of working theory with Korean emerging adults. *Journal of Counseling

Psychology, 66*(6), 701–713.

Kozan, S., Işık, E., & Blustein, D. L. (2019). Decent work and well-being among low-

income Turkish employees: Testing the psychology of working theory. *Journal of

Counseling Psychology, 66,* 317-327.

Kline, R. B. (2015). *Principles and practice of structural equation modeling.* New York,

NY: Guilford publications.

Krieger, N., Williams, D. R., & Moss, N. E. (1997). Measuring social class in US public

health research: Concepts, methodologies, and guidelines. *Annual Review of

Public Health, 18*(1), 341-378.

Krugman, P. (2012). *End this depression now!* New York, NY: WW Norton &

Company.

Lareau, A. (2011). *Unequal childhoods: Class, race, and family life*. Berkley, CA:

University of California Press.

Layte, R., & Maître, B. (2009). *The association between income inequality and mental

health: Social cohesion or social infrastructure?* (No. 328). ESRI Working Paper.

Lent, R. W. (2004). Toward a unifying theoretical and practical perspective on well-being

and psychosocial adjustment. *Journal of Counseling Psychology, 51*, 482–509.

Lent, R. W. (2013). Career-life preparedness: Revisiting career planning and adjustment

in the new workplace. *The Career Development Quarterly, 61*, 2–14.

Lewis, K. (2019). Making the connection: Transportation and youth disconnection. *Social

Science Research Council.*

Lim, C., & Sander, T. (2013). Does misery love company? Civic engagement in

economic hard times. *Social Science Research, 42*(1), 14-30.

Liu, W. M., Ali, S. R., Soleck, G., Hopps, J., Dunston, K., Pickett, T., & Hansen, J. C.

(2004). Using social class in counseling psychology research. *Journal of

Counseling Psychology, 51*(1), 3-18.

Metheny, J., & McWhirter, E. H. (2013). Contributions of social status and family

support to college students' career decision self-efficacy and outcome

expectations. *Journal of Career Assessment, 21*(3), 378-394.

MacLachlan, M. (2014). Macropsychology, policy, and global health. *American Psychologist, 69*(8), 851.

Marsh, H. W., Wen, Z., & Hau, K. (2004). Structural equation models of latent interactions: Evaluation of alternative estimation strategies and indicator construction. *Psychological Methods, 9,* 275-300.

Martens, M. P. (2005). The use of structural equation modeling in counseling psychology research. *The Counseling Psychologist, 33*(3), 296-298.

Mason, W., & Suri, S. (2012). Conducting behavioral research on Amazon's Mechanical Turk. *Behavior Research Methods, 44,* 1–23.

McDonald, R. P., & Ho, M. R. (2002). Principles and practice in reporting structural equation analyses. *Psychological Methods, 7*(1), 64-82.

McLaughlin, D. K., & Stokes, C. S. (2002). Income inequality and mortality in US counties: does minority racial concentration matter? *American journal of public health, 92*(1), 99-104.

Monnat, S. M. (2016). Deaths of Despair and Support for Trump in the 2016 Election. *The Pennsylvania State University Department of Agricultural Economics, Sociology, and Education Research Brief.* Retrieved from https://smmonnat.expressions.syr.edu/wp-content/uploads/ElectionBrief_DeathsofDespair.pdf

Monnat, S. M. (2018). Factors associated with county-level differences in US drug-related mortality rates. *American journal of preventive medicine, 54*(5), 611-619.

Monnat, S. M., & Brown, D. L. (2017). More than a Rural Revolt: Landscapes of Despair and the 2016 Presidential Election. *Journal of Rural Studies, 55,* 227-236.

Mouw, T., & Kalleberg, A. L. (2010). Occupations and the structure of wage inequality in the united states, 1980s to 2000s. *American Sociological Review, 75*(3), 402-431.

Muramatsu, N. (2003). County-level income inequality and depression among older Americans. *Health services research, 38*(6p2), 1863-1884.

Nussbaum, M. C. (2011). *Creating capabilities*. Cambridge, MA: Harvard University Press.

OECD. (2015). Securing livelihoods for all: Foresight for action. Development Centre Studies. Paris, France.

Patel, V., Burns, J. K., Dhingra, M., Tarver, L., Kohrt, B. A., & Lund, C. (2018). Income inequality and depression: a systematic review and meta-analysis of the association and a scoping review of mechanisms. *World Psychiatry, 17*(1), 76-89.

Paul, K. I., & Moser, K. (2009). Unemployment impairs mental health: Meta-analyses. *Journal of Vocational Behavior, 74*, 264–282.

Pavot, W. (2009). *Assessing well-being: The collected works of Ed Diener*. Dordrecht, Netherlands: Springer.

Piketty, T. (2014). Capital in the twenty-first century. Cambridge, MA: Harvard University Press.

Purdie-Vaughns, V., & Eibach, R. P. (2008). Intersectional invisibility: The distinctive advantages and disadvantages of multiple subordinate-group identities. *Sex Roles, 59*, 377–391.

Putnam, R. (2000). *Bowling alone: The collapse and revival of American community*. New York, NY: Simon & Schuster.

R Core Team (2020). *R: A language and environment for statistical computing*. R

Foundation for Statistical Computing, Vienna Austria. Retrieved from www.R-

project.org.

Revelle, W. (2019). *Psych: Procedures for personality and psychological research*.

Evanston, IL: Northwestern University. Retrieved from

www.CRAN.Rproject.org.

Richardson, M. S. (2000). A new perspective for counselors: From career ideologies to

empowerment through work and relationships practices. In A. Collin & R. Young

(Eds.), *The future of career* (pp. 197-211). New York, NY: Cambridge University

Press.

Robertson, P. J. (2015). Toward a capability approach to careers: Applying Amartya

Sen's thinking to career guidance and development. *International Journal of

Educational and Vocational Guidance, 15*, 75-88.

Roosa, M., Deng, S., Nair, R., & Burrell, G. (2005). Measures for studying poverty in

family and child research. *Journal of Marriage and Family, 67*, 971–988.

Rosseel, Y. (2012). Iavaan: An R package for structural equation modeling. *Journal of

Statistical Software, 48*(2), 1-36.

Sen, A. (1999). *Development as freedom*. New York, NY: Knopf.

Shah, A. K., Mullainathan, S., & Shafir, E. (2012). Some consequences of having too

little. *Science, 338*, 682-685.

Solar, O., & Irwin, A. (2018). A conceptual framework for action on the social

determinants of health. *Social Determinants of Health Discussion*. Paper 2 (Policy

and Practice).

Solberg, V. S. & Ali, S.R. (2017a). Career development research, practice, and policy: Synthesis and future directions. In V. S. Solberg & S. R. Ali (Eds.), *The Handbook of Career and Workforce Development: Research, Practice, and Policy* (pp, 243-264). New York, NY: Routledge.

Sharone, O. (2014). *Flawed system, flawed self: Job searching and unemployment experiences*. Chicago, IL: The University of Chicago Press.

Standing, G. (2010). *Work after globalization: Building occupational citizenship*. Cheltenham, United Kingdom: Edward Elgar.

Stiglitz, J. E. (2012). The price of inequality: How today's divided society endangers our future. New York, NY: Norton.

Stiglitz, J. (2015). *The great divide: Unequal societies and what we can do about them*. New York, NY: W. W. Norton.

Swanson, J. L. (2012). Work and psychological health. In N.A. Fouad, J. A Carter, & L. M. Subich (Eds.), *APA Handbook of Counseling Psychology, Vol. 2: Practice, interventions, and applications* (pp. 3-27). Washington, DC: American Psychological Association.

Swanson, J. L., Daniels, K. K., & Tokar, D. M. (1996). Assessing perceptions of career-related barriers: The career barriers inventory. *Journal of Career Assessment, 4,* 219–244.

U.S. Census Bureau (2017). American Community Survey. Retrieved from http://factfinder2.census.gov/faces/nav/jsf/pages/index.xhtml

Tabachnick, B. G., & Fidell, L. S. (2013). *Using multivariate statistics (6th ed.)*. Boston, MA: Pearson Education.

Thompson, M. N., & Dahling, J. J. (2010). Image theory and career aspirations: Indirect

and interactive effects of status-related variables. *Journal of Vocational Behavior,*

77, 21-29.

Thompson, M. N., & Subich, L. M. (2007). Exploration and validation of the Differential

Status Identity Scale. *Journal of Career Assessment, 15*(2), 227-239.

United State Bureau of Labor Statistics. (2020, May 12). *Employment projections:*

median age of labor force, by sex, race, and ethnicity. Retrieved from

https://www.bls.gov/emp/tables/median-age-labor-force.htm.

United States Census Bureau. (2020, May 30). Table 2. *Educational attainment of the*

population 25 years and over, by selected characteristics: 2019. Retrieved from

https://www.census.gov/data/tables/2019/demo/educational-attainment/cps-

detailedtables.html.

Wagmiller, R. L., & Adelman, R. M. (2009). Childhood and intergenerational poverty:

The long-term consequences of growing up poor. *National Center for Children in*

Poverty. Retrieved from http://hdl.handle.net/10022/AC:P:8870

Wang, D., Jia, Y., Hou, Zhi-Jin, Xu, H., Zhang, H., Guo, Z.L. (2019). A test of

psychology of working theory among Chinese urban workers: Examining

predictors and outcomes of decent work. *Journal of Vocational Behavior,* 115.

Weston, R., & Gore, P. A., Jr. (2006). A brief guide to structural equation modeling. *The*

Counseling Psychologist, 34, 719–751.

Wilmot, N. A., & Dauner, K. N. (2017). Examination of the influence of social capital on

depression in fragile families. *Journal of Epidemiology & Community*

Health, 71(3), 296-302.

Vallas, S. P. (2011). *Work: A critique*. Cambridge, United Kingdom: Polity.

Van Buuren, S. & Groothuis-Oudshoom, K. (2011). Mice: multivariate imputation by chained equations in R. *Journal of Statistical Software, 45*(3), 1-67.

Vinokur, A., Schul, Y., Vuori, J., & Price, R. (2000). Two years after a job loss: Long-term impact of the JOBS program on reemployment and mental health. *Journal of Occupational Health Psychology, 5*, 32–47.

Zimmerman, F. J., & Bell, J. F. (2006). Income inequality and physical and mental health: Testing associations consistent with proposed causal pathways. *Journal of Epidemiology & Community Health, 60*(6), 513-521.

Zoorob, M. J., & Salemi, J. L. (2017). Bowling alone, dying together: The role of social capital in mitigating the drug overdose epidemic in the United States. *Drug and alcohol dependence, 173*, 1-9.

Appendix A
Tables and Figures

Table A1
Regression coefficients for direct effects in full structural model with Five-factor decent work structure (N = 816)

Outcome regressed on predictor	B	SE	*t-value*	$P(>|t|)$	β
Life Satisfaction ~					
Safe	0.14	0.07	1.927	0.05	0.09
Healthcare	0.06	0.04	1.641	0.10	0.07
Compensation	0.16	0.05	3.427	0.00	0.16
Rest	-0.03	0.05	-0.557	0.58	-0.03
Values	0.26	0.05	4.919	0.00	0.23
Social Class	0.49	0.05	4.292	0.00	0.21
Safe ~					
Social Class	-0.08	0.10	-1.016	0.31	-0.05
Work Volition	0.48	0.05	9.159	0.00	0.56
Healthcare ~					
Social Class	0.70	0.12	5.955	0.00	0.25
Work Volition	0.63	0.06	9.775	0.00	0.42
Compensation ~					
Social Class	-0.05	0.11	-0.478	0.63	-0.02
Work Volition	0.58	0.07	8.554	0.00	0.48
Rest ~					
Social Class	-0.36	0.11	-3.245	0.00	-0.16
Work Volition	0.54	0.07	8.243	0.00	0.44
Values ~					
Social Class	0.04	0.08	0.539	0.60	0.02
Work Volition	0.74	0.05	14.975	0.00	0.66
Work Volition ~					
Social Class	0.82	0.10	8.083	0.00	0.44

Table A2
Regression coefficients for direct effects in full structural model with Bifactor decent work structure (N = 816)

Outcome regressed on predictor	B	SE	*t-value*	*P(>|t|)*	*β*
Life Satisfaction ~					
Safe	-0.10	0.08	-1.24	0.21	-0.06
Healthcare	-0.06	0.04	-1.52	0.13	-0.06
Compensation	0.06	0.05	1.24	0.22	0.06
Rest	-0.10	0.05	-2.09	0.04	-0.10
Values	-0.11	0.11	-0.99	0.32	-0.07
Social Class	0.10	0.13	0.74	0.46	0.04
DW	0.78	0.18	4.38	0.00	0.49
Safety ~					
Social Class	-0.25	0.12	-2.13	0.03	-0.20
Work Volition	-0.20	0.14	-1.45	0.15	-0.30
Healthcare ~					
Social Class	0.40	0.13	-2.13	0.03	-0.20
Work Volition	-0.32	0.14	-1.45	0.15	-0.30
Compensation ~					
Social Class	-0.32	0.19	-1.70	0.09	-0.16
Work Volition	-0.40	0.34	-1.19	0.24	-0.37
Rest ~					
Social Class	-0.55	0.21	-2.68	0.01	-0.26
Work Volition	-0.28	0.34	-0.81	0.42	-0.24
Values ~					
Social Class	-0.29	0.13	-2.28	0.02	-0.20
Work Volition	-0.31	0.12	-2.56	0.01	-0.41
Global Decent Work ~					
Social Class	0.25	0.10	2.45	0.01	0.17
Work Volition	0.62	0.14	4.50	0.00	0.79
Work Volition ~					
Social Class	0.81	0.10	8.71	0.00	0.46

Appendix B
Measures

Work Volition Scale: Volition subscale

Please select one answer to each of the following statements based on this scale.

Strongly Disagree (1)	Moderately Disagree (2)	Slightly Disagree (3)	Neutral (4)	Slightly Agree (5)	Moderately Agree (6)	Strongly Agree (7)

1) I've been able to choose the jobs I have wanted

2) I can do the kind of work I want, despite external barriers

3) I feel able to change jobs if I want to

4) I feel total control over my job choices.

Satisfaction with Life Scale

Below are five statements that you may agree or disagree with. Using the scale below, indicate your agreement with each item. Please be open and honest in your responding.

Strongly Agree (1)	Agree (2)	Slightly Agree (3)	Neither agree nor disagree (4)	Slightly disagree (5)	Disagree (6)	Strongly disagree (7)

1) In most ways my life is close to my ideal.

2) The conditions of my life are excellent.

3) I am satisfied with my life.

4) So far I have gotten the important things I want in life.

5) If I could live my life over, I would change almost nothing

Validity Check Question 1

Please select strongly agree on this statement

Strongly Disagree (1)	Moderately Disagree (2)	Slightly Disagree (3)	Neutral (4)	Slightly Agree (5)	Moderately Agree (6)	Strongly Agree (7)

Decent Work Scale

Please choose one answer to each of the following statements based on the scale.

Strongly Disagree (1)	Moderately Disagree (2)	Slightly Disagree (3)	Neutral (4)	Slightly Agree (5)	Moderately Agree (6)	Strongly Agree (7)

1) I feel emotionally safe interacting with people at work.

2) At work, I feel safe from emotional or verbal abuse of any kind.

3) I feel physically safe interacting with people at work.

4) I get good healthcare benefits from my job.

5) I have a good healthcare plan at work.

6) My employer provides acceptable options for healthcare.

7) I am not properly paid for my work. (reverse coded)

8) I do not feel I am paid enough based on my qualifications and experience. (reverse coded)

9) I am rewarded adequately for my work.

10) I do not have enough time for non-work activities. (reverse coded)

11) I have no time to rest during the work week. (reverse coded)

12) I have free time during the work week.

13) The values of my organization match my family values.

14) My organization's values align with my family values.

15) The values of my organization match the values within my community.

Validity Check Question 2

Please select disagree on this statement

Strongly Disagree (1)	Moderately Disagree (2)	Slightly Disagree (3)	Neutral (4)	Slightly Agree (5)	Moderately Agree (6)	Strongly Agree (7)

Demographic Questions

Please tell us a little about yourself. This information will be used only to describe the sample as a group.

What is your age?

____

How would you identify your gender? If your identity is not captured fully with these categories, please feel free to specify further.

○ Man

○ Woman

○ Transgender

○ Other ____

What is your race/ethnicity? (You may select more than one)

○ African/African-American/Black

○ American Indian/Native American/First Nation

○ Arab American/Middle Eastern

○ Asian/Asian American

○ Asian Indian

○ Hispanic/Latina/o American

○ Pacific Islander

○ White/European American/Caucasian

○ Other _______________________________________

Highest degree obtained?

- ○ Less than High School (1)
- ○ Some High School (2)
- ○ High School Graduate (3)
- ○ Trade/Vocational School (4)
- ○ Some College (5)
- ○ College Degree (e.g. B. A., B.S.) (6)
- ○ Professional Degree (e.g., M.B.A., M.S., Ph.D, M.D., etc.) (7)

What is your average yearly household income?

- ○ Less than $25,000 per year
- ○ $25,000-$50,000 per year
- ○ $51,000-$75,000 per year
- ○ $76,000-$100,000 per year
- ○ $101,000-$125,000 per year
- ○ $126,000-$150,000 per year
- ○ $151,000-$175,000 per year
- ○ $176,000-$200,000 per year
- ○ $201,000 + per year
- ○ I don't know

How would you identify your current social class?

○ Lower class

○ Working class

○ Middle class

○ Upper middle class

○ Upper class

How would you identify your childhood social class?

○ Lower class

○ Working class

○ Middle class

○ Upper middle class

○ Upper class

Validity Check Question 3

Did you take this survey seriously?

○ Yes

○ No

2017 Opportunity Index Data Sources

The indicators that comprise the 2017 Opportunity Index are derived from a number of sources - Census Bureau data and statistics compiled by reputable nonprofit organizations.

Economy
Indicator: Unemployment rate
Definition: The total number of people without jobs who actively looked for work within the preceding four weeks and were available to take a job, as a percentage of the total number in the labor force (those working or unemployed).
Source: Bureau of Labor Statistics, Local Area Unemployment Statistics and news releases (http://www.bls.gov/lau/)
Note: Rates in the 2017 Opportunity Index refer to April 2017 and are not seasonally adjusted.

Indicator: Median household income
Definition: The income level that falls at the midpoint of the total distribution of households, ranked from richest to poorest. Household income includes work earnings from jobs or self employment, as well as income from interest, dividends, rent, Social Security, pension payments, unemployment compensation, cash welfare benefits and other forms of money regularly received by any member of the household.
Source: U.S. Census Bureau, American Community Survey (http://factfinder2.census.gov/faces/nav/jsf/pages/index.xhtml).
Note: Because income is not distributed evenly across households, the average (mean) is much higher than the median, and thus the median is generally considered to give a fairer picture of income for a "typical" household. In the 2017 Opportunity Index, median household income data at the state level refer to 2015; for counties, data refer to 2011–2015. To facilitate year-to-year comparisons, income figures presented in the Opportunity Index are adjusted for inflation so they can be expressed in 2010 doll

Indicator: Poverty rate
Definition: Percentage of people of all ages living with family incomes below the federal poverty line.
Source: U.S. Census Bureau, American Community Survey
(http://factfinder2.census.gov/faces/nav/jsf/pages/index.xhtml).
Note: The federal poverty line is the amount of pretax cash income considered adequate for an individual or family to meet basic needs. It is updated annually for inflation, based on Consumer Price Index changes, and is adjusted for family size and composition. In 2015, a four-person family with two children would be considered to live in poverty if it had income less than $24,046. Poverty rate data in the 2017 Opportunity Index for states and the nation refer to 2015; county data refer to 2011–2015.

Indicator: 80/20 ratio (ratio of household income at the 80th percentile of income to that of the 20th percentile)
Definition: The 80/20 ratio is a measure of income inequality describing the disparity in income between the household at the 80th percentile of income and the household at the 20th percentile. The 80/20 ratio for the United States is 4.9, meaning that the wealthiest fifth of households (those at the 20th percentile) have incomes nearly five times higher than those of households in the poorest fifth (the 80th percentile).
Source: U.S. Census Bureau, American Community Survey
(http://factfinder2.census.gov/faces/nav/jsf/pages/index.xhtml).
Note: 80/20 ratio data in the 2017 Opportunity Index for states and the nation refer to 2015 income; data for counties use 2011–2015 income.

Indicator: Number of banking institutions (commercial banks, savings institutions and credit unions) per 10,000 residents
Definition: The number of commercial banks, savings institutions and credit unions per 10,000 residents.
Source: Child Trends' analysis of data from the U.S. Census Bureau, County Business Patterns
(https://www.census.gov/programs-surveys/cbp.html) and Population Estimates
(https://www.census.gov/programs- surveys/popest.html).
Note: Banking institutions included in this indicator include those under the following NAICS codes: 522110, 522120 and 522130. In the 2017 Opportunity Index, data for this indicator refer to 2015.

Indicator: Households spending less than 30 percent of household income on housing-related costs
Definition: The percentage of households spending less than 30 percent of their income on rent and utilities (for households who rent), or on mortgage payments and other housing-related costs, such as real estate taxes or condo fees (for those who own homes).
Source: U.S. Census Bureau, American Community Survey
(http://factfinder2.census.gov/faces/nav/jsf/pages/index.xhtml).
Note: A widely accepted cut-off for housing affordability is housing-related costs that are no more than 30 percent of household income. Housing units for which costs and/or household income could not be determined are excluded from the calculation. For the nation and states, data refer to 2015; data for counties refer to 2011–2015.

Indicator: Broadband internet subscription
Definition: The percentage of households with subscriptions to broadband internet service (including both cable and DSL internet).
Source: U.S. Census Bureau, American Community Survey
(http://factfinder2.census.gov/faces/nav/jsf/pages/index.xhtml)
Note: This indicator is new to the 2017 Opportunity Index, replacing the percentage of households with high-speed internet—for which data are no longer collected. Broadband internet data in the 2017 Opportunity Index are from 2015. In the updated 2016 Index, data refer to 2014.

<u>Education</u>
Indicator: Preschool enrollment
Definition: The percentage of children ages three and four enrolled in public or private nursery school, preschool or kindergarten.
Source: U.S. Census Bureau, American Community Survey
(http://factfinder2.census.gov/faces/nav/jsf/pages/index.xhtml).
Note: Data on preschool enrollment for states and the nation refer to 2015; data for counties refer to 2011–2015.

Indicator: On-time high school graduation rate
Definition: The percentage of high school freshmen who graduate after four years of high school.
Source: National and state data are from EDFacts' Adjusted Cohort

Graduation Rate (ACGR) (https://www2.ed.gov/about/inits/ed/edfacts/data- files/index.html); county data are taken from the Robert Wood Johnson Foundation's County Health Rankings' analysis of school district-level ACGR data from the EDFacts site (http://www.countyhealthrankings.org/ resources/2017-chr-measures-data-sources-and-years).

Note: The ACGR is calculated as "the number of students who graduate in four years with a regular high school diploma, divided by the number of students who form the adjusted cohort of the graduating class. From the beginning of 9th grade (or the earliest high school grade), students who are entering that grade for the first time make up a cohort that is 'adjusted' by adding any students who subsequently transfer into the cohort and subtracting any students who subsequently transfer out, emigrate to another country or die."[1] Data for this indicator refer to the 2014–2015 school year.

Prior to 2015, the Opportunity Index used a different measure, the Average Freshmen Graduation Rate, that is not comparable to the ACGR. The Department of Education stopped updating the Average Freshman Graduation Rate in 2012, adopting the ACGR as their preference, which is the indicator used in the Index since 2015.

Indicator: Associate degree or higher
Definition: The percentage of adults ages 25 and older who have completed an associate degree or higher.
Source: U.S. Census Bureau, American Community Survey (http://factfinder2.census.gov/faces/nav/jsf/pages/index.xhtml).
Note: Data for states and the nation refer to 2015; county-level data refer to 2011–2015.

Health
Indicator: Low birth weight
Definition: The percentage of live births where the infant weighed less than 2,500 grams (approximately 5 lbs., 8 oz.).
Source: CDC WONDER (https://wonder.cdc.gov/natality-current.html) **Note:** This indicator is new to the 2017 Opportunity Index. Data for states and the nation refer to 2015; data for counties refer to 2011–2015. The updated 2016 Index also includes this indicator; data for states and the

---

[1] U.S. Department of Education. (2015). *Regulatory Four-Year Adjusted Cohort Graduation Rates - School Year 2013-14, EDFacts Data Documentation.* Washington, DC: U.S. Department of Education. Retrieved from http://www.ed.gov/edfacts.

nation refer to 2014; data for counties refer to 2010–2014.

Indicator: Health insurance
Definition: The percentage of the population under age 65 not covered by health insurance.
Source: American Community Survey
(http://factfinder2.census.gov/faces/nav/jsf/pages/index.xhtml)
Note: This indicator is new to the 2017 Opportunity Index. Data for states and the nation refer to 2015; data for counties refer to 2011–2015. The updated 2016 Index also includes this indicator; data for states and the nation refer to 2014; data for counties refer to 2010–2014.

Indicator: Deaths related to alcohol/drug use or suicide (rate per 100,000) **Definition:** The age-adjusted number of deaths, per 100,000 population, due to poisoning from drugs (including recreational and prescription drugs), or alcohol, or suicide.
Source: CDC WONDER (https://wonder.cdc.gov/ucd-icd10.html)
Note: This indicator is new to the 2017 Opportunity Index. The calculation includes several reported underlying causes of death compiled by CDC Wonder. The following ICD-10 codes are included: X40-X45, X60-X84 and Y10-Y15. Age adjusting accounts for localities differing in their age composition. Data for states and the nation refer to 2015; data for counties refer to 2011–2015. The updated 2016 Index also includes this indicator; data for states and the nation refer to 2014; data for counties refer to 2010–2014.

<u>**Community**</u>
Indicator: Volunteering
Definition: The percentage of adults ages 18 and older who performed volunteer work through or for an organization at any time in the previous year.
Source: Child Trends' analysis of data from the U.S. Census Bureau, Current Population Survey and Volunteering Supplement. Due to sample-size limitations of the survey data, this indicator is calculated at the national and state levels only.
Note: Two years of survey responses were pooled to increase the sample available for analysis. This makes for more stable estimates.

This indicator was updated slightly for the 2017 Opportunity Index and draws from two survey questions: "Since September 1 of last year, have you done any volunteer activities through or for an organization?" and "Sometimes people don't think of activities they do infrequently or activities they do for children's schools or youth organizations as volunteer activities. Since September 1 of last year, have you done any of these types of volunteer activities?" Data in the 2017 Opportunity Index refer to 2014– 2015. The updated 2016 Index also draws from these survey questions; data refer to 2013–2014.

Prior to 2016, this indicator relied on the single question, "Since September 1 of last year, have you done any volunteer activities through or for an organization?"

Indicator: Voter registration rate
Definition: The percentage of the adult population registered to vote. **Source:** U.S. Census Bureau, Voting and Registration (https://www.census.gov/data/tables/time-series/demo/voting-and- registration/p20-580.html)
Note: This indicator is new to the 2017 Opportunity Index. Historically, voter registration is higher in presidential election years than in midterm election years. This indicator will be updated biannually so that each update provides a rolling average that includes the most recent presidential election year and midterm election year. Data in the 2017 Opportunity Index are the average of registration rates for 2014 and 2016. The updated 2016 Index also includes this indicator; data are the average of registration rates in 2012 and 2014. Because counties and congressional districts frequently follow different borders, this indicator is calculated at the national and state levels only.

Indicator: Youth not in school and not working
Definition: The percentage of the population ages 16 to 24 who are not enrolled in school and not working or not currently seeking employment. **Source:** Child Trends' analysis of data from the U.S. Census Bureau, American Community Survey, PUMS Microdata (https://www.census.gov/programs-surveys/acs/data/pums.html) and custom tabulations for county and county equivalents provided by special arrangement with the U.S. Census Bureau.
Note: Data in the 2017 Opportunity Index for states and the nation refer to

2015; data for counties refer to 2011–2015.

Indicator: Violent crime rate
Definition: Total number of violent crimes reported to local law enforcement agencies, per 100,000 people. Violent crimes include homicide, rape, robbery and assault.
Source: State and national data are from the U.S. Department of Justice, Federal Bureau of Investigation Uniform Crime Reporting, Crime in the U.S. (https://ucr.fbi.gov/crime-in-the-u.s/); county data from the County Health Rankings analysis of data from the U.S. Department of Justice, Federal Bureau of Investigation Criminal Justice Information Services. County Health Rankings is a project of the University of Wisconsin Population Health Institute in collaboration with the Robert Wood Johnson Foundation. Crime data are based on report data provided by nearly 17,000 law enforcement agencies (LEAs) across the United States. Due to the number of reporting agencies, there is a reporting lag; not all LEAs report and some data reported may be incomplete.
Note: Data in the 2017 Opportunity Index for states and the nation refer to 2015; data for counties refer to 2012–2014.

Indicator: Primary care physicians
Definition: Number of primary care physicians per 100,000 population. **Source:** Bureau of Health Workforce, Area Health Resources Files (https://datawarehouse.hrsa.gov/data/datadownload.aspx)
Note: This indicator is new to the 2017 Opportunity Index, replacing an indicator calculated as the number of doctors per 100,000 population. Data in the 2017 Opportunity Index refer to 2015. The updated 2016 Index also includes this indicator; data refer to 2014. State and national statistics for this indicator are derived from the county-level Area Health Resources Files. The number of primary care physicians includes non-federal physicians who are not currently in a residency program and who are younger than age 75.

Indicator: Grocery stores and produce vendors
Definition: The number of supermarkets, grocery stores and produce stands per 10,000 residents.
Source: Child Trends' analysis of data from the U.S. Census Bureau, County Business Patterns and Population Estimates Program (http://www.census.gov/econ/cbp/index.html and

http://www.census.gov/popest/).
Note: NAICS codes 445110 and 445230 are used to gather the number of supermarkets, grocery stores and produce stands. Data in the 2017 Opportunity Index refer to 2015.

Indicator: Incarceration rate
Definition: The number of people incarcerated in jails or prisons per 100,000 residents ages 18 and older.
Source: Bureau of Justice Statistics, Correctional Populations in the United States (https://www.bjs.gov/index.cfm?ty=tp&tid=11).
Note: This indicator is new to the 2017 Opportunity Index. Data are available at the national and state level only. Data in the 2017 Opportunity Index refer to 2015. The updated 2016 Opportunity Index also includes this indicator; data refer to 20

Opportunity Index Methodology

The Opportunity Index draws upon statistics from a variety of sources, including the U.S. Census Bureau, U.S. Department of Labor Statistics and the U.S. Department of Justice. Calculating Opportunity Scores for states and grades for counties entails three steps:

1. Rescaling indicators
2. Calculating dimension scores
3. Calculating Opportunity Scores and Grades

Rescaling Indicators

The diverse indicators that comprise the Opportunity Index include percentages, rates and dollar values. To include them in a composite measure such as the Opportunity Index, we transform each of these statistics to enable comparisons on a common scale. The Opportunity Index uses a simple rescaling procedure based on the minimum and maximum values obtained for each indicator.[2]

Each state or county's performance on an indicator is compared with the highest and lowest scores obtained on that indicator, excluding outliers (extreme values).[3] The following formula is used to calculate a value from 0 to 100 for each indicator:

$$\text{Observed value rescaled} = \left(\frac{\text{Observed value} - \text{Lowest value}}{\text{Highest value} - \text{Lowest value}} \times 100 \right)$$

The indicators in the Opportunity Index vary in their directionality. For example, median household income is an indicator for which higher values are more desirable, but the unemployment rate is better when lower.

---

[2] The natural logs of the data for median household income and violent crime are used in this process to normalize their highly skewed data distributions.

[3] The maximum and minimum values for each indicator are based on an examination of variance and skewness.

For indicators with long tails on either or both sides of the normal distribution curve, maximum and minimum values are set to fall within the long tails, with values outside of this range treated as equivalent to the minimum or maximum in the rescaling process.

For negative indicators,[4] the rescaling procedure also standardizes their directionality:

$$\text{Observed value rescaled} = 1 - \left(\frac{\text{Observed value} - \text{Lowest value}}{\text{Highest value} - \text{Lowest value}} \right) \times 100$$

This way, for all indicators, higher values are more desirable. The highest and lowest values for each indicator are presented below:

Economy

INDICATOR	DESCRIPTION	LOWEST VALUE	HIGHEST VALUE
JOBS	Unemployment rate (percentage of the population ages 16 and older who are not working and are seeking work and available to work)	0.0	**16.0**
WAGES	Median household income (in 2010 dollars)	$19,000	$95,000
POVERTY	Percentage of the population below the federal poverty level	2.0	30.0
INCOME INEQUALITY	80/20 ratio (ratio of household income at the 80th percentile to that at the 20th percentile)	2.0	7.0
ACCESS TO BANKING SERVICES	Number of banking institutions (commercial banks, savings institutions and credit unions) per 10,000 residents	0.0	10.5
AFFORDABLE HOUSING	Percentage of households spending less than 30 percent of their income on housing-related costs	40.0	95.0
BROADBAND INTERNET SUBSCRIPTION	Percentage of households with subscriptions to broadband internet service	50.0	100.0

Education

INDICATOR	DESCRIPTION	LOWEST VALUE	HIGHEST VALUE
PRESCHOOL ENROLLMENT	Percentage of 3- and 4-year-olds attending preschool	0.0	100.0
HIGH SCHOOL GRADUATIO N	On-time high school graduation rate (percentage of freshmen who graduate in four years)	55.0	100.0
POSTSECONDAR Y EDUCATION	Percentage of adults ages 25 and older with an associate's degree or higher	0.0	75.0

Health

INDICATOR	DESCRIPTION	LOWEST VALUE	HIGHEST VALUE
LOW BIRTH WEIGHT	Percentage of infants born weighing less than 5.5 pounds	4.0	11.5
HEALTH INSURANCE COVERAGE	Percentage of the population (under age 65) without health insurance coverage	0.0	30.0
DEATHS RELATED TO ALCOHOL / DRUG USE AND SUICIDE	Deaths attributed to alcohol or drug poisoning, or suicide (age-adjusted rate per 100,000 population)	0.0	60.0

Community

INDICATOR	DESCRIPTION	LOWEST VALUE	HIGHEST VALUE
VOLUNTEERING	Percentage of adults (ages 18 and older) who reported volunteering during the previous year **[national and state-level only]**	0.0	65.0
VOTER REGISTRATIO N	Percentage of the population ages 18 and older who are registered to vote **[national and state-level only]**	35.0	90.0
YOUTH DISCONNECTION	Percentage of youth ages 16–24 not in school and not working	0.0	30.0

VIOLENT CRIME	Incidents of violent crime reported to law enforcement agencies (per 100,000 population)	0.0	12.0
ACCESS TO PRIMARY HEALTH CARE	Number of primary care physicians (per 100,000 population)	0.0	175.0
ACCESS TO HEALTHY FOOD	Number of grocery stores and produce vendors (per 10,000 population)	0.0	6.3
INCARCERATION	Number of people incarcerated in jail or prison (per 100,000 population ages 15–64) **[national and state-level only]**	300.0	1500.0

Calculating Dimension Scores

At the state level, the Opportunity Index is made up of 20 indicators across the four dimensions (Economy, Education, Health and Community). In each dimension, the rescaled values for indicators are averaged to create dimension-level Opportunity Scores, also ranging from 1 to 100. Because data for some indicators are not available at the county level,[5] the county Opportunity Index is made up of 17 indicators. As with states, indicators in each dimension are averaged to create dimension-level Opportunity Scores ranging from 0 to 100.

Calculating Opportunity Scores and Grades

Each state also has an overall Opportunity Score that summarizes performance across the four Index dimensions. To calculate these, a state's four dimension scores are averaged with equal weighting. Final Opportunity Scores are again represented as values from 0 to 100; these values are used to rank the 50 states and the District of Columbia on the Opportunity Index. To create overall county Opportunity Scores, the four dimension scores are again averaged and weighted equally. Counties are also assigned Opportunity Grades that correspond to their scores, ranging from A+ to F.

In 2011, Opportunity Grade cut-off points were based on the distribution of raw, final numerical outcomes of the 2011 Opportunity Index for counties and county equivalents; groupings were done by standard deviations above or below the average. The same cut-off points were used to assign Opportunity Grades for the 2012 to 2016 indices, allowing comparison across years.

However, in 2017, it was necessary to recalculate the relationship between final numerical values and Opportunity Grade assignments because of the significant update to the dimensions and indicators comprising the Opportunity Index. New cut-off points for assigning grades were based on the distribution of numerical scores of the updated Opportunity Index in 2016 for counties and county equivalents. Grades in the 2017 Index were also assigned according to these new cut-off points. Thus, it is valid to compare county grades between the updated 2016 and 2017 indices.
However, Opportunity Grades from 2011 to 2015 were based on the 2011 cut-off points. Because of this, county grades from 2011 to 2015 (or from the original 2016 Index) should not be compared with those from the updated 2016 Index or 2017 Index.

The assignment of county-level Opportunity Grades based on the standardized scores is summarized in the table below.

Opportunity Grade	Minimum Standardized Score (rounded)	Maximum Standardized Score (rounded)
A+	80.0	100.0
A	67.5	79.9
A-	64.0	67.4
B+	60.5	63.9
B	57.1	60.4
B-	53.6	57.0
C+	50.1	53.5
C	46.6	50.0
C-	43.1	46.5

D+	39.6	43.0
D	36.2	39.7
D-	32.7	36.1
F	0.0	32.6

Data Notes

Given the large number of geographic areas and the many indicators that comprise the Opportunity Index, it is not surprising that there are instances of missing data. If a county is missing data for more than two indicators, or for two or more indicators within the same dimension, then an Opportunity Grade is not calculated for that county.[6] If a county is missing data for one or two indicators, with a maximum of one missing indicator per dimension, then the rescaled state average is substituted for the missing data point. Of a total of 3,142 counties and county equivalents, 1,085 counties were excluded from the 2017 Opportunity Index due to missing or unreliable data. Missing data was highest for the low birth weight and broadband internet indicators.

Most indicators in the Opportunity Index are based on survey data; thus, they are statistical estimates and may be subject to sampling and non- sampling error. Therefore, differences in dimension scores, Opportunity Scores and Opportunity Grades between different geographic areas and across different years are not necessarily statistically significant, and comparisons should be made with caution.

Correlations and Internal Consistency

Correlations

The updates included in the 2017 Opportunity Index call for a re- examination of how well its component indicators "hang together" as a single measure of opportunity. One way to do this is to examine the correlation between each rescaled indicator and the overall Opportunity Score.[7] Correlation values can range between -1.0 and 1.0.

In 2017, the indicators most closely related to overall opportunity were the incarceration rate (at the state level only), with a correlation of 0.82, and the percentage of the population with an associate degree or higher, with a correlation of 0.78. The indicator least closely related to overall opportunity was the percentage of households spending less than 30 percent of their income on housing costs; this indicator was negatively associated with overall opportunity.

All of the dimension scores were strongly related to overall opportunity; Health had the strongest correlation, at 0.84. Other notable findings were strong correlations between Health and Economy (0.60), between Health and Community (0.51), between Health and Education (0.50) and between Education and Community (0.55). Detailed results from correlation analyses are presented below.

Dimension Score Correlations: All Dimensions and Overall Opportunity Score				
	Dimension Scores				Opportunity Score
	Economy	Education	Health	Community	Opportunity Score
Economy	-	0.50	0.60	0.43	0.79
Education	0.50	-	0.50	0.55	0.78
Health	0.60	0.50	-	0.51	0.84
Community	0.43	0.55	0.51	-	0.78